TABLE OF CONTENTS

Top 20 Test Taking Tips

1. Carefully follow all the test registration procedures
2. Know the test directions, duration, topics, question types, how many questions
3. Setup a flexible study schedule at least 3-4 weeks before test day
4. Study during the time of day you are most alert, relaxed, and stress free
5. Maximize your learning style; visual learner use visual study aids, auditory learner use auditory study aids
6. Focus on your weakest knowledge base
7. Find a study partner to review with and help clarify questions
8. Practice, practice, practice
9. Get a good night's sleep; don't try to cram the night before the test
10. Eat a well balanced meal
11. Know the exact physical location of the testing site; drive the route to the site prior to test day
12. Bring a set of ear plugs; the testing center could be noisy
13. Wear comfortable, loose fitting, layered clothing to the testing center; prepare for it to be either cold or hot during the test
14. Bring at least 2 current forms of ID to the testing center
15. Arrive to the test early; be prepared to wait and be patient
16. Eliminate the obviously wrong answer choices, then guess the first remaining choice
17. Pace yourself; don't rush, but keep working and move on if you get stuck
18. Maintain a positive attitude even if the test is going poorly
19. Keep your first answer unless you are positive it is wrong
20. Check your work, don't make a careless mistake

Verbal Test Review

The Verbal test of the RN Pre-entrance Exam consists of a total of 60 questions in two categories: Word Knowledge and Reading Comprehension.

Word Knowledge

Determining Word Meaning

An understanding of the basics of language is helpful, and often vital, to understanding what you read. The term *structural analysis* refers to looking at the parts of a word and breaking it down into its different components to determine the word's meaning. Parts of a word include prefixes, suffixes, and the root word. By learning the meanings of prefixes, suffixes, and other word fundamentals, you can decipher the meaning of words which may not yet be in your vocabulary. Prefixes are common letter combinations at the beginning of words, while suffixes are common letter combinations at the end. The main part of the word is known as the root. Visually, it would look like this: prefix + root word + suffix. Look first at the individual meanings of the root word, prefix and/or suffix. Using knowledge of the meaning(s) of the prefix and/or suffix to see what information it adds to the root. Even if the meaning of the root is unknown, one can use knowledge of the prefix's and/or suffix's meaning(s) to determine an approximate meaning of the word. For example, if one sees the word *uninspired* and does not know what it means, they can use the knowledge that *un-* means 'not' to know that the full word means "not inspired." Understanding the common prefixes and suffixes can illuminate at least part of the meaning of an unfamiliar word.

Below is a list of common prefixes and their meanings:

Prefix	Definition	Examples
a	in, on, of, up, to	abed, afoot
a-	without, lacking	atheist, agnostic
ab-	from, away, off	abdicate, abjure
ad-	to, toward	advance
am-	friend, love	amicable, amatory
ante-	before, previous	antecedent, antedate
anti-	against, opposing	antipathy, antidote
auto-	self	autonomy, autobiography
belli-	war, warlike	bellicose
bene-	well, good	benefit, benefactor
bi-	two	bisect, biennial
bio-	life	biology, biosphere
cata-	down, away, thoroughly	catastrophe, cataclysm
chron-	time	chronometer, synchronize
circum-	around	circumspect, circumference

com-	with, together, very	commotion, complicate
contra-	against, opposing	contradict, contravene
cred-	belief, trust	credible, credit
de-	from	depart
dem-	people	demographics, democracy
dia-	through, across, apart	diameter, diagnose
dis-	away, off, down, not	dissent, disappear
epi-	upon	epilogue
equi-	equal, equally	equivalent
ex-	out	extract
for-	away, off, from	forget, forswear
fore-	before, previous	foretell, forefathers
homo-	same, equal	homogenized
hyper-	excessive, over	hypercritical, hypertension
hypo-	under, beneath	hypodermic, hypothesis
in-	in, into	intrude, invade
in-	not, opposing	incapable, ineligible
inter-	among, between	intercede, interrupt
intra-	within	intramural, intrastate
magn-	large	magnitude, magnify
mal-	bad, poorly, not	malfunction
micr-	small	microbe, microscope
mis-	bad, poorly, not	misspell, misfire
mono-	one, single	monogamy, monologue
mor-	die, death	mortality, mortuary
neo-	new	neolithic, neoconservative
non-	not	nonentity, nonsense
ob-	against, opposing	objection
omni-	all, everywhere	omniscient
ortho-	right, straight	orthogonal, orthodox
over-	above	overbearing
pan-	all, entire	panorama, pandemonium
para-	beside, beyond	parallel, paradox
per-	through	perceive, permit
peri-	around	periscope, perimeter
phil-	love, like	philosophy, philanthropic
poly-	many	polymorphous, polygamous
post-	after, following	postpone, postscript
pre-	before, previous	prevent, preclude
prim-	first, early	primitive, primary
pro-	forward, in place of	propel, pronoun
re-	back, backward, again	revoke, recur
retro-	back, backward	retrospect, retrograde
semi-	half, partly	semicircle, semicolon

sub-	under, beneath	subjugate, substitute
super-	above, extra	supersede, supernumerary
sym-	with, together	sympathy, symphony
trans-	across, beyond, over	transact, transport
ultra-	beyond, excessively	ultramodern, ultrasonic, ultraviolet
un-	not, reverse of	unhappy, unlock
uni-	one	uniform, unity
vis-	to see	visage, visible

Below is a list of common suffixes and their meanings:

Suffix	Definition	Examples
-able	able to, likely	capable, tolerable
-age	process, state, rank	passage, bondage
-ance	act, condition, fact	acceptance, vigilance
-arch	to rule	monarch
-ard	one that does excessively	drunkard, wizard
-ate	having, showing	separate, desolate
-ation	action, state, result	occupation, starvation
-cy	state, condition	accuracy, captaincy
-dom	state, rank, condition	serfdom, wisdom
-en	cause to be, become	deepen, strengthen
-er	one who does	teacher
-esce	become, grow, continue	convalesce, acquiesce
-esque	in the style of, like	picturesque, grotesque
-ess	feminine	waitress, lioness
-fic	making, causing	terrific, beatific
-ful	full of, marked by	thankful, zestful
-fy	make, cause, cause to have	glorify, fortify
-hood	state, condition	manhood, statehood
-ible	able, likely, fit	edible, possible, divisible
-ion	action, result, state	union, fusion
-ish	suggesting, like	churlish, childish
-ism	act, manner, doctrine	barbarism, socialism
-ist	doer, believer	monopolist, socialist
-ition	action, state, result	sedition, expedition
-ity	state, quality, condition	acidity, civility
-ize	make, cause to be, treat with	sterilize, mechanize, criticize
-less	lacking, without	hopeless, countless
-like	like, similar	childlike, dreamlike
-logue	type of written/spoken language	prologue
-ly	like, of the nature of	friendly, positively
-ment	means, result, action	refreshment, disappointment
-ness	quality, state	greatness, tallness

-or	doer, office, action	juror, elevator, honor
-ous	marked by, given to	religious, riotous
-ship	the art or skill of	statesmanship
-some	apt to, showing	tiresome, lonesome
-th	act, state, quality	warmth, width
-tude	quality, state, result	magnitude, fortitude
-ty	quality, state	enmity, activity
-ward	in the direction of	backward, homeward

When defining words in a text, words often have a meaning that is more than the dictionary definition. The **denotative** meaning of a word is the literal meaning. The **connotative** meaning goes beyond the denotative meaning to include the emotional reaction a word may invoke. The connotative meaning often takes the denotative meaning a step further due to associations which the reader makes with the denotative meaning. The reader can differentiate between the denotative and connotative meanings by first recognizing when authors use each meaning. Most non-fiction, for example, is fact-based, the authors not using flowery, figurative language. The reader can assume that the writer is using the denotative, or literal, meaning of words. In fiction, on the other hand, the author may be using the connotative meaning. Connotation is one form of figurative language. The reader should use context clues to determine if the author is using the denotative or connotative meaning of a word.

> ➤ **Review Video: <u>Denotative and Connotative Meaning</u>**
> *Visit **mometrix.com/academy** and enter **Code: 736707***

Readers of all levels will encounter words with which they are somewhat unfamiliar. The best way to define a word in **context** is to look for nearby words that can help. For instance, unfamiliar nouns are often accompanied by examples that furnish a definition. Consider the following sentence: "Dave arrived at the party in hilarious garb: a leopard-print shirt, buckskin trousers, and high heels." If a reader was unfamiliar with the meaning of garb, he could read the examples and quickly determine that the word means "clothing." Examples will not always be this obvious. For instance, consider this sentence: "Parsley, lemon, and flowers were just a few of items he used as garnishes." Here, the possibly unfamiliar word *garnishes* is exemplified by parsley, lemon, and flowers. Readers who have eaten in a few restaurants will probably be able to identify a garnish as something used to decorate a plate.

> ➤ **Review Video: <u>Context</u>**
> *Visit **mometrix.com/academy** and enter **Code: 613660***

In addition to looking at the context of a passage, readers can often use contrasts to define an unfamiliar word in context. In many sentences, the author will not describe the unfamiliar word directly, but will instead describe the opposite of the

- *10* -

unfamiliar word. Of course, this provides information about the word the reader needs to define. Consider the following example: "Despite his intelligence, Hector's low brow and bad posture made him look obtuse." The author suggests that Hector's appearance was opposite to his actual intelligence. Therefore, *obtuse* must mean unintelligent or stupid. Here is another example: "Despite the horrible weather, we were beatific about our trip to Alaska." The word *despite* indicates that the speaker's feelings were at odds with the weather. Since the weather is described as "horrible," *beatific* must mean something good.

In some cases, there will be very few contextual clues to help a reader define the meaning of an unfamiliar word. When this happens, one strategy the reader may employ is substitution. A good reader will brainstorm some possible synonyms for the given word, and then substitute these words into the sentence. If the sentence and the surrounding passage continue to make sense, the substitution has revealed at least some information about the unfamiliar word. Consider the sentence, "Frank's admonition rang in her ears as she climbed the mountain." A reader unfamiliar with *admonition* might come up with some substitutions like "vow," "promise," "advice," "complaint," or "compliment." All of these words make general sense of the sentence, though their meanings are diverse. The process has suggested, however, that an admonition is some sort of message. The substitution strategy is rarely able to pinpoint a precise definition, but can be effective as a last resort.

It is sometimes possible to define an unfamiliar word by looking at the descriptive words in the context. Consider the following sentence: "Fred dragged the recalcitrant boy kicking and screaming up the stairs." *Dragged*, *kicking*, and *screaming* all suggest that the boy does not want to go up the stairs. The reader may assume that *recalcitrant* means something like unwilling or protesting. In that example, an unfamiliar adjective was identified. It is perhaps more typical to use description to define an unfamiliar noun, as in this sentence: "Don's wrinkled frown and constantly shaking fist identified him as a curmudgeon of the first order." Don is described as having a "wrinkled frown and constantly shaking fist," suggesting that a *curmudgeon* must be a grumpy old man. Contrasts do not always provide detailed information about the unfamiliar word, but they at least give the reader some clues.

When a word has more than one meaning, it can be tricky to determine how it is being used in a given sentence. Consider the verb *cleave*, which bizarrely can mean either "join" or "separate." When a reader comes upon this word, she will have to select the definition that makes the most sense. So, take as an example the following sentence: "The birds cleaved together as they flew from the oak tree." Immediately, the presence of the word *together* should suggest that in this sentence *cleave* is being used to mean "*join*." A slightly more difficult example would be the sentence, "Hermione's knife cleaved the bread cleanly." It doesn't make sense for a knife to join bread together, so the word must be meant to indicate separation. Discovering the meaning of a word with multiple meanings requires the same tricks as defining an unknown word: looking for contextual clues and evaluating substituted words.

Nearly and Perfect Synonyms

You must determine which of four provided choices has the best similar definition as a certain word. Nearly similar may often be more correct, because the goal is to test your understanding of the nuances, or little differences, between words. A perfect match may not exist, so don't be concerned if your answer choice is not a complete synonym. Focus upon edging closer to the word. Eliminate the words that you know aren't correct first. Then narrow your search. Cross out the words that are the least similar to the main word until you are left with the one that is the most similar.

Prefixes

Take advantage of every clue that the word might include. Prefixes and suffixes can be a huge help. Usually they allow you to determine a basic meaning. Pre- means before, post- means after, pro – is positive, de- is negative. From these prefixes and suffixes, you can get an idea of the general meaning of the word and look for its opposite. Beware though of any traps. Just because con is the opposite of pro, doesn't necessarily mean congress is the opposite of progress! A list of the most common prefixes and suffixes is included in a special report at the end.

Positive vs. Negative

Many words can be easily determined to be a positive word or a negative word. Words such as despicable, gruesome, and bleak are all negative. Words such as ecstatic, praiseworthy, and magnificent are all positive. You will be surprised at how many words can be considered as either positive or negative. Once that is determined, you can quickly eliminate any other words with an opposite meaning and focus on those that have the other characteristic, whether positive or negative.

Word Strength

Part of the challenge is determining the most nearly similar word. This is particularly true when two words seem to be similar. When analyzing a word, determine how strong it is. For example, stupendous and good are both positive words. However, stupendous is a much stronger positive adjective than good. Also, towering or gigantic are stronger words than tall or large. Search for an answer choice that is similar and also has the same strength. If the main word is weak, look for similar words that are also weak. If the main word is strong, look for similar words that are also strong.

Type and Topic

Another key is what type of word is the main word. If the main word is an adjective describing height, then look for the answer to be an adjective describing height as well. Match both the type and topic of the main word. The type refers the parts of speech, whether the word is an adjective, adverb, or verb. The topic refers to what the definition of the word includes, such as sizes or fashion styles.

Form a Sentence

Many words seem more natural in a sentence. *Specious* reasoning, *irresistible* force, and *uncanny* resemblance are just a few of the word combinations that usually go together. When faced with an uncommon word that you barely understand (and on the RN Pre-entrance exam there will be many), try to put the word in a sentence that makes sense. It will help you to understand the word's meaning and make it easier to determine its opposite. Once you have a good descriptive sentence that utilizes the main word properly, plug in the answer choices and see if the sentence still has the same meaning with each answer choice. The answer choice that maintains the meaning of the sentence is correct!

Use Replacements

Using a sentence is a great help because it puts the word into a proper perspective. Since the RN Pre-entrance exam actually gives you a sentence, sometimes you don't always have to create your own (though in many cases the sentence won't be helpful). Read the provided sentence, picking out the main word. Then read the sentence again and again, each time replacing the main word with one of the answer choices. The correct answer should "sound" right and fit.
Example: The desert landscape was desolate. Desolate means
    A. cheerful
    B. creepy
    C. excited
    D. forlorn
After reading the example sentence, begin replacing "desolate" with each of the answer choices. Does "the desert landscape was cheerful, creepy, excited, or forlorn" sound right? Deserts are typically hot, empty, and rugged environments, probably not cheerful, or excited. While creepy might sound right, that word would certainly be more appropriate for a haunted house. But "the desert landscape was forlorn" has a certain ring to it and would be correct.

Eliminate Similar Choices

If you don't know the word, don't worry. Look at the answer choices and just use them. Remember that three of the answer choices will always be wrong. If you can find a common relationship between any three answer choices, then you know they are wrong. Find the answer choice that does not have a common relationship to the other answer choices and it will be the correct answer.
Example: Laconic most nearly means
    A. wordy
    B. talkative
    C. expressive
    D. quiet
In this example the first three choices are all similar. Even if you don't know that laconic means the same as quiet, you know that "quiet" must be correct, because the other three choices were all virtually the same. They were all the same, so they

must all be wrong. The one that is different must be correct. So, don't worry if you don't know a word. Focus on the answer choices that you do understand and see if you can identify similarities. Even identifying two words that are similar will allow you to eliminate those two answer choices, for they are both wrong, because they are either both right or both wrong (they're similar, remember), so since they can't both be right, they both must be wrong.

Example:
He worked slowly, moving the leather back and forth until it was ____ .
    A. rough
    B. hard
    C. stiff
    D. pliable

In this example the first three choices are all similar and synonyms. Even without knowing what pliable means, it has to be correct, because you know the other three answer choices mean the same thing.

Adjectives Give it Away
Words mean things and are added to the sentence for a reason. Adjectives in particular may be the clue to determining which answer choice is correct.
Example:
The brilliant scientist made several discoveries that were
    A. dull
    B. dazzling
Look at the adjectives first to help determine what makes sense. A "brilliant" or smart scientist would make dazzling, rather than dull discoveries. Without that simple adjective, no answer choice is clear.

Use Logic
Ask yourself questions about each answer choice to see if they are logical.
Example:
In the distance, the deep pounding resonance of the drums could be
    A. seen
    B. heard
Would resonating poundings be "seen"? or Would resonating pounding be "heard"?

The Trap of Familiarity
Don't just choose a word because you recognize it. On difficult questions, you may only recognize one or two words. The RN Pre-entrance exam doesn't put "make-believe words" on the test, so don't think that just because you only recognize one word means that word must be correct. If you don't recognize four words, then focus on the one that you do recognize. Is it correct? Try your best to determine if it fits the sentence. If it does, that is great, but if it doesn't, eliminate it.

Reading Comprehension

Comprehension Skills

One of the most important skills in reading comprehension is the identification of **topics** and **main ideas.** There is a subtle difference between these two features. The topic is the subject of a text, or what the text is about. The main idea, on the other hand, is the most important point being made by the author. The topic is usually expressed in a few words at the most, while the main idea often needs a full sentence to be completely defined. As an example, a short passage might have the topic of penguins and the main idea *Penguins are different from other birds in many ways.* In most nonfiction writing, the topic and the main idea will be stated directly, often in a sentence at the very beginning or end of the text. When being tested on an understanding of the author's topic, the reader can quickly *skim* the passage for the general idea, stopping to read only the first sentence of each paragraph. A paragraph's first sentence is often (but not always) the main topic sentence, and it gives you a summary of the content of the paragraph. However, there are cases in which the reader must figure out an unstated topic or main idea. In these instances, the student must read every sentence of the text, and try to come up with an overarching idea that is supported by each of those sentences.

> ➤ **Review Video: Topics and Main Ideas**
> *Visit **mometrix.com/academy** and enter **Code: 407801***

While the main idea is the overall premise of a story, **supporting details** provide evidence and backing for the main point. In order to show that a main idea is correct, or valid, the author needs to add details that prove their point. All texts contain details, but they are only classified as supporting details when they serve to reinforce some larger point. Supporting details are most commonly found in informative and persuasive texts. In some cases, they will be clearly indicated with words like *for example* or *for instance*, or they will be enumerated with words like *first*, *second*, and *last*. However, they may not be indicated with special words. As a reader, it is important to consider whether the author's supporting details really back up his or her main point. Supporting details can be factual and correct but still not relevant to the author's point. Conversely, supporting details can seem pertinent but be ineffective because they are based on opinion or assertions that cannot be proven.

> ➤ **Review Video: Supporting Details**
> *Visit **mometrix.com/academy** and enter **Code: 396297***

An example of a main idea is: "Giraffes live in the Serengeti of Africa." A supporting detail about giraffes could be: "A giraffe uses its long neck to reach twigs and leaves on trees." The main idea gives the general idea that the text is about giraffes. The supporting detail gives a specific fact about how the giraffes eat.

As opposed to a main idea, themes are seldom expressed directly in a text, so they can be difficult to identify. A **theme** is an issue, an idea, or a question raised by the text. For instance, a theme of William Shakespeare's *Hamlet* is indecision, as the title character explores his own psyche and the results of his failure to make bold choices. A great work of literature may have many themes, and the reader is justified in identifying any for which he or she can find support. One common characteristic of themes is that they raise more questions than they answer. In a good piece of fiction, the author is not always trying to convince the reader, but is instead trying to elevate the reader's perspective and encourage him to consider the themes more deeply. When reading, one can identify themes by constantly asking what general issues the text is addressing. A good way to evaluate an author's approach to a theme is to begin reading with a question in mind (for example, how does this text approach the theme of love?) and then look for evidence in the text that addresses that question.

> ➢ **Review Video:** <u>Theme</u>
> *Visit **mometrix.com/academy** and enter **Code:** **732074***

Purposes for Writing
In order to be an effective reader, one must pay attention to the author's **position** and purpose. Even those texts that seem objective and impartial, like textbooks, have some sort of position and bias. Readers need to take these positions into account when considering the author's message. When an author uses emotional language or clearly favors one side of an argument, his position is clear. However, the author's position may be evident not only in what he writes, but in what he doesn't write. For this reason, it is sometimes necessary to review some other texts on the same topic in order to develop a view of the author's position. If this is not possible, then it may be useful to acquire a little background personal information about the author. When the only source of information is the text, however, the reader should look for language and argumentation that seems to indicate a particular stance on the subject.

Identifying the **purpose** of an author is usually easier than identifying her position. In most cases, the author has no interest in hiding his or her purpose. A text that is meant to entertain, for instance, should be obviously written to please the reader. Most narratives, or stories, are written to entertain, though they may also inform or persuade. Informative texts are easy to identify as well. The most difficult purpose of a text to identify is persuasion, because the author has an interest in making this purpose hard to detect. When a person knows that the author is trying to convince him, he is automatically more wary and skeptical of the argument.

For this reason persuasive texts often try to establish an entertaining tone, hoping to amuse the reader into agreement, or an informative tone, hoping to create an appearance of authority and objectivity.

> ➢ **Review Video: <u>Purpose of an Author</u>**
> *Visit **mometrix.com/academy** and enter **Code: 497555***

An author's purpose is often evident in the organization of the text. For instance, if the text has headings and subheadings, if key terms are in bold, and if the author makes his main idea clear from the beginning, then the likely purpose of the text is to inform. If the author begins by making a claim and then makes various arguments to support that claim, the purpose is probably to persuade. If the author is telling a story, or is more interested in holding the attention of the reader than in making a particular point or delivering information, then his purpose is most likely to entertain. As a reader, it is best to judge an author on how well he accomplishes his purpose. In other words, it is not entirely fair to complain that a textbook is boring: if the text is clear and easy to understand, then the author has done his job. Similarly, a storyteller should not be judged too harshly for getting some facts wrong, so long as he is able to give pleasure to the reader.

The author's purpose for writing will affect his writing style and the response of the reader. In a **persuasive essay**, the author is attempting to change the reader's mind or convince him of something he did not believe previously. There are several identifying characteristics of persuasive writing. One is opinion presented as fact. When an author attempts to persuade the reader, he often presents his or her opinions as if they were fact. A reader must be on guard for statements that sound factual but which cannot be subjected to research, observation, or experiment. Another characteristic of persuasive writing is emotional language. An author will often try to play on the reader's emotion by appealing to his sympathy or sense of morality. When an author uses colorful or evocative language with the intent of arousing the reader's passions, it is likely that he is attempting to persuade. Finally, in many cases a persuasive text will give an unfair explanation of opposing positions, if these positions are mentioned at all.

> ➢ **Review Video: <u>Persuasive Essay</u>**
> *Visit **mometrix.com/academy** and enter **Code: 621428***

An **informative text** is written to educate and enlighten the reader. Informative texts are almost always nonfiction, and are rarely structured as a story. The intention of an informative text is to deliver information in the most comprehensible way possible, so the structure of the text is likely to be very clear. In an informative text, the thesis statement is often in the first sentence. The author may use some colorful language, but is likely to put more emphasis on clarity and precision. Informative essays do not typically appeal to the emotions. They often contain facts and figures, and rarely include the opinion of the author. Sometimes a

- 17 -

persuasive essay can resemble an informative essay, especially if the author maintains an even tone and presents his or her views as if they were established fact.

➢ **Review Video: Informative Text**
Visit mometrix.com/academy and enter Code: **924964**

The success or failure of an author's intent to **entertain** is determined by those who read the author's work. Entertaining texts may be either fiction or nonfiction, and they may describe real or imagined people, places, and events. Entertaining texts are often narratives, or stories. A text that is written to entertain is likely to contain colorful language that engages the imagination and the emotions. Such writing often features a great deal of figurative language, which typically enlivens its subject matter with images and analogies. Though an entertaining text is not usually written to persuade or inform, it may accomplish both of these tasks. An entertaining text may appeal to the reader's emotions and cause him or her to think differently about a particular subject. In any case, entertaining texts tend to showcase the personality of the author more so than do other types of writing.

When an author intends to **express feelings,** she may use colorful and evocative language. An author may write emotionally for any number of reasons. Sometimes, the author will do so because she is describing a personal situation of great pain or happiness. Sometimes an author is attempting to persuade the reader, and so will use emotion to stir up the passions. It can be easy to identify this kind of expression when the writer uses phrases like *I felt* and *I sense.* However, sometimes the author will simply describe feelings without introducing them. As a reader, it is important to recognize when an author is expressing emotion, and not to become overwhelmed by sympathy or passion. A reader should maintain some detachment so that he or she can still evaluate the strength of the author's argument or the quality of the writing.

➢ **Review Video: Express Feelings**
Visit mometrix.com/academy and enter Code: **759390**

In a sense, almost all writing is descriptive, insofar as it seeks to describe events, ideas, or people to the reader. Some texts, however, are primarily concerned with **description**. A descriptive text focuses on a particular subject, and attempts to depict it in a way that will be clear to the reader. Descriptive texts contain many adjectives and adverbs, words that give shades of meaning and create a more detailed mental picture for the reader. A descriptive text fails when it is unclear or vague to the reader. On the other hand, however, a descriptive text that compiles too much detail can be boring and overwhelming to the reader.

A descriptive text will certainly be informative, and it may be persuasive and entertaining as well. Descriptive writing is a challenge for the author, but when it is done well, it can be fun to read.

- 18 -

Writing Devices

Authors will use different stylistic and writing devices to make their meaning more clearly understood. One of those devices is comparison and contrast. When an author describes the ways in which two things are alike, he or she is **comparing** them. When the author describes the ways in which two things are different, he or she is **contrasting** them. The "compare and contrast" essay is one of the most common forms in nonfiction. It is often signaled with certain words: a comparison may be indicated with such words as *both*, *same*, *like*, *too*, and *as well*; while a contrast may be indicated by words like *but*, *however*, *on the other hand*, *instead*, and *yet*. Of course, comparisons and contrasts may be implicit without using any such signaling language. A single sentence may both compare and contrast. Consider the sentence *Brian and Sheila love ice cream, but Brian prefers vanilla and Sheila prefers strawberry*. In one sentence, the author has described both a similarity (love of ice cream) and a difference (favorite flavor).

> ➤ **Review Video: <u>Compare and Contrast</u>**
> *Visit **mometrix.com/academy** and enter **Code: 798319***

One of the most common text structures is **cause and effect**. A cause is an act or event that makes something happen, and an effect is the thing that happens as a result of that cause. A cause-and-effect relationship is not always explicit, but there are some words in English that signal causality, such as *since*, *because*, and *as a result*. As an example, consider the sentence *Because the sky was clear, Ron did not bring an umbrella*. The cause is the clear sky, and the effect is that Ron did not bring an umbrella. However, sometimes the cause-and-effect relationship will not be clearly noted. For instance, the sentence *He was late and missed the meeting* does not contain any signaling words, but it still contains a cause (he was late) and an effect (he missed the meeting). It is possible for a single cause to have multiple effects, or for a single effect to have multiple causes. Also, an effect can in turn be the cause of another effect, in what is known as a cause-and-effect chain.

Authors often use analogies to add meaning to the text. An **analogy** is a comparison of two things. The words in the analogy are connected by a certain, often undetermined relationship. Look at this analogy: moo is to cow as quack is to duck. This analogy compares the sound that a cow makes with the sound that a duck makes. Even if the word 'quack' was not given, one could figure out it is the correct word to complete the analogy based on the relationship between the words 'moo' and 'cow'. Some common relationships for analogies include synonyms, antonyms, part to whole, definition, and actor to action.

Another element that impacts a text is the author's point of view. The **point of view** of a text is the perspective from which it is told. The author will always have a point of view about a story before he draws up a plot line. The author will know what events they want to take place, how they want the characters to interact, and how the story will resolve. An author will also have an opinion on the topic, or series of events, which is presented in the story, based on their own prior experience and beliefs.

➢ **Review Video: <u>Point of View</u>**
*Visit **mometrix.com/academy** and enter **Code:** 383336*

The two main points of view that authors use are first person and third person. If the narrator of the story is also the main character, or *protagonist*, the text is written in first-person point of view. In first person, the author writes with the word *I.* Third-person point of view is probably the most common point of view that authors use. Using third person, authors refer to each character using the words *he* or *she.* In third-person omniscient, the narrator is not a character in the story and tells the story of all of the characters at the same time.

A good writer will use **transitional words** and phrases to guide the reader through the text. You are no doubt familiar with the common transitions, though you may never have considered how they operate. Some transitional phrases (*after, before, during, in the middle of*) give information about time. Some indicate that an example is about to be given (*for example, in fact, for instance*). Writers use them to compare (*also, likewise*) and contrast (*however, but, yet*). Transitional words and phrases can suggest addition (*and, also, furthermore, moreover*) and logical relationships (*if, then, therefore, as a result, since*). Finally, transitional words and phrases can demarcate the steps in a process (*first, second, last*). You should incorporate transitional words and phrases where they will orient your reader and illuminate the structure of your composition.

➢ **Review Video: <u>Transitional Words and Phrases</u>**
*Visit **mometrix.com/academy** and enter **Code:** 197796*

Types of Passages

A **narrative** passage is a story. Narratives can be fiction or nonfiction. However, there are a few elements that a text must have in order to be classified as a narrative. To begin with, the text must have a plot. That is, it must describe a series of events. If it is a good narrative, these events will be interesting and emotionally engaging to the reader. A narrative also has characters. These could be people, animals, or even inanimate objects, so long as they participate in the plot. A narrative passage often contains figurative language, which is meant to stimulate the imagination of the reader by making comparisons and observations. A metaphor, which is a description of one thing in terms of another, is a common piece of figurative language. *The moon was a frosty snowball* is an example of a metaphor: it is obviously untrue in the literal sense, but it suggests a certain mood for the reader. Narratives often proceed in a clear sequence, but they do not need to do so.

➢ **Review Video: <u>Narratives</u>**
*Visit **mometrix.com/academy** and enter **Code:** 280100*

An **expository** passage aims to inform and enlighten the reader. It is nonfiction and usually centers around a simple, easily defined topic. Since the goal of exposition is to teach, such a passage should be as clear as possible. It is common for an expository passage to contain helpful organizing words, like *first, next, for example*, and *therefore*. These words keep the reader oriented in the text. Although expository passages do not need to feature colorful language and artful writing, they are often more effective when they do. For a reader, the challenge of expository passages is to maintain steady attention. Expository passages are not always about subjects in which a reader will naturally be interested, and the writer is often more concerned with clarity and comprehensibility than with engaging the reader. For this reason, many expository passages are dull. Making notes is a good way to maintain focus when reading an expository passage.

> ➢ **Review Video: <u>Expository Passages</u>**
> *Visit **mometrix.com/academy** and enter **Code: 256515***

A **technical** passage is written to describe a complex object or process. Technical writing is common in medical and technological fields, in which complicated mathematical, scientific, and engineering ideas need to be explained simply and clearly. To ease comprehension, a technical passage usually proceeds in a very logical order. Technical passages often have clear headings and subheadings, which are used to keep the reader oriented in the text. It is also common for these passages to break sections up with numbers or letters. Many technical passages look more like an outline than a piece of prose. The amount of jargon or difficult vocabulary will vary in a technical passage depending on the intended audience. As much as possible, technical passages try to avoid language that the reader will have to research in order to understand the message. Of course, it is not always possible to avoid jargon.

A **persuasive** passage is meant to change the reader's mind or lead her into agreement with the author. The persuasive intent may be obvious, or it may be quite difficult to discern. In some cases, a persuasive passage will be indistinguishable from an informative passage: it will make an assertion and offer supporting details. However, a persuasive passage is more likely to make claims based on opinion and to appeal to the reader's emotions. Persuasive passages may not describe alternate positions and, when they do, they often display significant bias. It may be clear that a persuasive passage is giving the author's viewpoint, or the passage may adopt a seemingly objective tone. A persuasive passage is successful if it can make a convincing argument and win the trust of the reader.

A persuasive essay will likely focus on one central argument, but it may make many smaller claims along the way. These are subordinate arguments with which the reader must agree if he or she is going to agree with the central argument. The central argument will only be as strong as the subordinate claims. These claims

- *21* -

should be rooted in fact and observation, rather than subjective judgment. The best persuasive essays provide enough supporting detail to justify claims without overwhelming the reader. Remember that a fact must be susceptible to independent verification: that is, it must be something the reader could confirm. Also, statistics are only effective when they take into account possible objections. For instance, a statistic on the number of foreclosed houses would only be useful if it was taken over a defined interval and in a defined area. Most readers are wary of statistics, because they are so often misleading. If possible, a persuasive essay should always include references so that the reader can obtain more information. Of course, this means that the writer's accuracy and fairness may be judged by the inquiring reader.

Opinions are formed by emotion as well as reason, and persuasive writers often appeal to the feelings of the reader. Although readers should always be skeptical of this technique, it is often used in a proper and ethical manner. For instance, there are many subjects that have an obvious emotional component, and therefore cannot be completely treated without an appeal to the emotions. Consider an article on drunk driving: it makes sense to include some specific examples that will alarm or sadden the reader. After all, drunk driving often has serious and tragic consequences. Emotional appeals are not appropriate, however, when they attempt to mislead the reader. For instance, in political advertisements it is common to emphasize the patriotism of the preferred candidate, because this will encourage the audience to link their own positive feelings about the country with their opinion of the candidate. However, these ads often imply that the other candidate is unpatriotic, which in most cases is far from the truth. Another common and improper emotional appeal is the use of loaded language, as for instance referring to an avidly religious person as a "fanatic" or a passionate environmentalist as a "tree hugger." These terms introduce an emotional component that detracts from the argument.

> **Review Video: Persuasive Techniques**
> *Visit **mometrix.com/academy** and enter **Code: 577997***

History and Culture
Historical context has a profound influence on literature: the events, knowledge base, and assumptions of an author's time color every aspect of his or her work. Sometimes, authors hold opinions and use language that would be considered inappropriate or immoral in a modern setting, but that was acceptable in the author's time. As a reader, one should consider how the historical context influenced a work and also how today's opinions and ideas shape the way modern readers read the works of the past. For instance, in most societies of the past, women were treated as second-class citizens. An author who wrote in 18th-century England might sound sexist to modern readers, even if that author was relatively feminist in his time. Readers should not have to excuse the faulty assumptions and prejudices of the past, but they should appreciate that a person's thoughts and words are, in

part, a result of the time and culture in which they live or lived, and it is perhaps unfair to expect writers to avoid all of the errors of their times.

➤ **Review Video: Historical Context**
Visit ***mometrix.com/academy*** *and enter* ***Code:*** **169770**

Even a brief study of world literature suggests that writers from vastly different cultures address similar themes. For instance, works like the *Odyssey* and *Hamlet* both tackle the individual's battle for self-control and independence. In every culture, authors address themes of personal growth and the struggle for maturity. Another universal theme is the conflict between the individual and society. In works as culturally disparate as *Native Son*, the *Aeneid*, and *1984*, authors dramatize how people struggle to maintain their personalities and dignity in large, sometimes oppressive groups. Finally, many cultures have versions of the hero's (or heroine's) journey, in which an adventurous person must overcome many obstacles in order to gain greater knowledge, power, and perspective. Some famous works that treat this theme are the *Epic of Gilgamesh*, Dante's *Divine Comedy*, and *Don Quixote.*

Authors from different genres (for instance poetry, drama, novel, short story) and cultures may address similar themes, but they often do so quite differently. For instance, poets are likely to address subject matter obliquely, through the use of images and allusions. In a play, on the other hand, the author is more likely to dramatize themes by using characters to express opposing viewpoints. This disparity is known as a dialectical approach. In a novel, the author does not need to express themes directly; rather, they can be illustrated through events and actions. In some regional literatures, like those of Greece or England, authors use more irony: their works have characters that express views and make decisions that are clearly disapproved of by the author. In Latin America, there is a great tradition of using supernatural events to illustrate themes about real life. In China and Japan, authors frequently use well-established regional forms (haiku, for instance) to organize their treatment of universal themes.

Responding to Literature
When reading good literature, the reader is moved to engage actively in the text. One part of being an active reader involves making predictions. A **prediction** is a guess about what will happen next. Readers are constantly making predictions based on what they have read and what they already know. Consider the following sentence: *Staring at the computer screen in shock, Kim blindly reached over for the brimming glass of water on the shelf to her side.* The sentence suggests that Kim is agitated and that she is not looking at the glass she is going to pick up, so a reader might predict that she is going to knock the glass over.

Of course, not every prediction will be accurate: perhaps Kim will pick the glass up cleanly. Nevertheless, the author has certainly created the expectation that the water might be spilled. Predictions are always subject to revision as the reader acquires more information.

> **Review Video: Prediction**
> Visit *mometrix.com/academy* and enter *Code: 437248*

Test-taking tip: To respond to questions requiring future predictions, the student's answers should be based on evidence of past or present behavior.

Readers are often required to understand text that claims and suggests ideas without stating them directly. An **inference** is a piece of information that is implied but not written outright by the author. For instance, consider the following sentence: *Mark made more money that week than he had in the previous year*. From this sentence, the reader can infer that Mark either has not made much money in the previous year or made a great deal of money that week. Often, a reader can use information he or she already knows to make inferences. Take as an example the sentence *When his coffee arrived, he looked around the table for the silver cup*. Many people know that cream is typically served in a silver cup, so using their own base of knowledge they can infer that the subject of this sentence takes his coffee with cream. Making inferences requires concentration, attention, and practice.

> **Review Video: Inference**
> Visit *mometrix.com/academy* and enter *Code: 379203*

Test-taking tip: While being tested on his ability to make correct inferences, the student must look for contextual clues. An answer can be *true* but not *correct*. The contextual clues will help you find the answer that is the best answer out of the given choices. Understand the context in which a phrase is stated. When asked for the implied meaning of a statement made in the passage, the student should immediately locate the statement and read the context in which it was made. Also, look for an answer choice that has a similar phrase to the statement in question.

A reader must be able to identify a text's **sequence**, or the order in which things happen. Often, and especially when the sequence is very important to the author, it is indicated with signal words like *first*, *then*, *next*, and *last*. However, sometimes a sequence is merely implied and must be noted by the reader. Consider the sentence *He walked in the front door and switched on the hall lamp*. Clearly, the man did not turn the lamp on before he walked in the door, so the implied sequence is that he first walked in the door and then turned on the lamp. Texts do not always proceed in an orderly sequence from first to last: sometimes, they begin at the end and then start over at the beginning. As a reader, it can be useful to make brief notes to clarify the sequence.

> **Review Video: Sequence**
> Visit *mometrix.com/academy* and enter *Code: 489027*

In addition to inferring and predicting things about the text, the reader must often **draw conclusions** about the information he has read. When asked for a *conclusion* that may be drawn, look for critical "hedge" phrases, such as *likely, may, can, will often,* among many others. When you are being tested on this knowledge, remember that question writers insert these hedge phrases to cover every possibility. Often an answer will be wrong simply because it leaves no room for exception. Extreme positive or negative answers (such as always, never, etc.) are usually not correct. The reader should not use any outside knowledge that is not gathered from the reading passage to answer the related questions. Correct answers can be derived straight from the reading passage.

Literary Genres

Literary genres refer to the basic generic types of poetry, drama, fiction, and nonfiction. Literary genre is a method of classifying and analyzing literature. There are numerous subdivisions within genre, including such categories as novels, novellas, and short stories in fiction. Drama may also be subdivided into comedy, tragedy, and many other categories. Poetry and nonfiction have their own distinct divisions.

Genres often overlap, and the distinctions among them are blurred, such as that between the nonfiction novel and docudrama, as well as many others. However, the use of genres is helpful to the reader as a set of understandings that guide our responses to a work. The generic norm sets expectations and forms the framework within which we read and evaluate a work. This framework will guide both our understanding and interpretation of the work. It is a useful tool for both literary criticism and analysis.

Fiction is a general term for any form of literary narrative that is invented or imagined rather than being factual. For those individuals who equate fact with truth, the imagined or invented character of fiction tends to render it relatively unimportant or trivial among the genres. Defenders of fiction are quick to point out that the fictional mode is an essential part of being. The ability to imagine or discuss what-if plots, characters, and events is clearly part of the human experience.

Prose is derived from the Latin and means "straightforward discourse." Prose fiction, although having many categories, may be divided into three main groups:
- **Short stories**: a fictional narrative, the length of which varies, usually under 20,000 words. Short stories usually have only a few characters and generally describe one major event or insight. The short story began in magazines in the late 1800s and has flourished ever since.
- **Novels**: a longer work of fiction, often containing a large cast of characters and extensive plotting. The emphasis may be on an event, action, social problems, or any experience. There is now a genre of nonfiction novels pioneered by Truman Capote's *In Cold Blood* in the 1960s. Novels may also be written in verse.

- **Novellas**: a work of narrative fiction longer than a short story but shorter than a novel. Novellas may also be called short novels or novelettes. They originated from the German tradition and have become common forms in all of the world's literature.

Many elements influence a work of prose fiction. Some important ones are:
- Speech and dialogue: Characters may speak for themselves or through the narrator. Dialogue may be realistic or fantastic, depending on the author's aim.
- Thoughts and mental processes: There may be internal dialogue used as a device for plot development or character understanding.
- Dramatic involvement: Some narrators encourage readers to become involved in the events of the story, whereas others attempt to distance readers through literary devices.
- Action: This is any information that advances the plot or involves new interactions between the characters.
- Duration: The time frame of the work may be long or short, and the relationship between described time and narrative time may vary.
- Setting and description: Is the setting critical to the plot or characters? How are the action scenes described?
- Themes: This is any point of view or topic given sustained attention.
- Symbolism: Authors often veil meanings through imagery and other literary constructions.

Fiction is much wider than simply prose fiction. Songs, ballads, epics, and narrative poems are examples of non-prose fiction. A full definition of fiction must include not only the work itself but also the framework in which it is read. Literary fiction can also be defined as not true rather than nonexistent, as many works of historical fiction refer to real people, places, and events that are treated imaginatively as if they were true. These imaginary elements enrich and broaden literary expression.

When analyzing fiction, it is important for the reader to look carefully at the work being studied. The plot or action of a narrative can become so entertaining that the language of the work is ignored. The language of fiction should not simply be a way to relate a plot—it should also yield many insights to the judicious reader. Some prose fiction is based on the reader's engagement with the language rather than the story. A studious reader will analyze the mode of expression as well as the narrative. Part of the reward of reading in this manner is to discover how the author uses different language to describe familiar objects, events, or emotions. Some works focus the reader on an author's unorthodox use of language, whereas others may emphasize characters or storylines. What happens in a story is not always the critical element in the work. This type of reading may be difficult at first but yields great rewards.

The **narrator** is a central part of any work of fiction, and can give insight about the purpose of the work and its main themes and ideas. The following are important questions to address to better understand the voice and role of the narrator and incorporate that voice into an overall understanding of the novel:

- Who is the narrator of the novel? What is the narrator's perspective, first person or third person? What is the role of the narrator in the plot? Are there changes in narrators or the perspective of narrators?
- Does the narrator explain things in the novel, or does meaning emerge from the plot and events? The personality of the narrator is important. She may have a vested interest in a character or event described. Some narratives follow the time sequence of the plot, whereas others do not. A narrator may express approval or disapproval about a character or events in the work.
- Tone is an important aspect of the narration. Who is actually being addressed by the narrator? Is the tone familiar or formal, intimate or impersonal? Does the vocabulary suggest clues about the narrator?

> ➢ **Review Video: The Narrator**
> *Visit **mometrix.com/academy** and enter **Code: 742528***

A **character** is a person intimately involved with the plot and development of the novel. Development of the novel's characters not only moves the story along but will also tell the reader a lot about the novel itself. There is usually a physical description of the character, but this is often omitted in modern and postmodern novels. These works may focus on the psychological state or motivation of the character. The choice of a character's name may give valuable clues to his role in the work.

Characters are said to be flat or round. Flat characters tend to be minor figures in the story, changing little or not at all. Round characters (those understood from a well-rounded view) are more central to the story and tend to change as the plot unfolds. Stock characters are similar to flat characters, filling out the story without influencing it.

Modern literature has been greatly affected by Freudian psychology, giving rise to such devices as the interior monologue and magical realism as methods of understanding characters in a work. These give the reader a more complex understanding of the inner lives of the characters and enrich the understanding of relationships between characters.

> ➢ **Review Video: Characters**
> *Visit **mometrix.com/academy** and enter **Code: 429493***

Another important genre is that of **drama**: a play written to be spoken aloud. The drama is in many ways inseparable from performance. Reading drama ideally involves using imagination to visualize and re-create the play with characters and settings. The reader stages the play in his imagination, watching characters interact and developments unfold. Sometimes this involves simulating a theatrical presentation; other times it involves imagining the events. In either case, the reader is imagining the unwritten to re-create the dramatic experience. Novels present some of the same problems, but a narrator will provide much more information about the setting, characters, inner dialogues, and many other supporting details. In drama, much of this is missing, and we are required to use our powers of projection and imagination to taste the full flavor of the dramatic work. There are many empty spaces in dramatic texts that must be filled by the reader to fully appreciate the work.

> ➤ **Review Video: <u>Dramas</u>**
> *Visit **mometrix.com/academy** and enter **Code: 216060***

When reading drama in this way, there are some advantages over watching the play performed (though there is much criticism in this regard):

- Freedom of point of view and perspective: Text is free of interpretations of actors, directors, producers, and technical staging.
- Additional information: The text of a drama may be accompanied by notes or prefaces placing the work in a social or historical context. Stage directions may also provide relevant information about the author's purpose. None of this is typically available at live or filmed performances.
- Study and understanding: Difficult or obscure passages may be studied at leisure and supplemented by explanatory works. This is particularly true of older plays with unfamiliar language, which cannot be fully understood without an opportunity to study the material.

Critical elements of drama, especially when it is being read aloud or performed, include dialect, speech, and dialogue. Analysis of speech and dialogue is important in the critical study of drama. Some playwrights use speech to develop their characters. Speeches may be long or short, and written in as normal prose or blank verse. Some characters have a unique way of speaking which illuminates aspects of the drama. Emphasis and tone are both important, as well. Does the author make clear the tone in which lines are to be spoken, or is this open to interpretation? Sometimes there are various possibilities in tone with regard to delivering lines.

Dialect is any distinct variety of a language, especially one spoken in a region or part of a country. The criterion for distinguishing dialects from languages is that of mutual understanding. For example, people who speak Dutch cannot understand English unless they have learned it. But a speaker from Amsterdam can understand one from Antwerp; therefore, they speak different dialects of the same language. This is, however, a matter of degree; there are languages in which different dialects are unintelligible.

Dialect mixtures are the presence in one form of speech with elements from different neighboring dialects. The study of speech differences from one geographical area to another is called dialect geography. A dialect atlas is a map showing distribution of dialects in a given area. A dialect continuum shows a progressive shift in dialects across a territory, such that adjacent dialects are understandable, but those at the extremes are not.

Dramatic dialogue can be difficult to interpret and changes depending upon the tone used and which words are emphasized. Where the stresses, or meters, of dramatic dialogue fall can determine meaning. Variations in emphasis are only one factor in the manipulability of dramatic speech. Tone is of equal or greater importance and expresses a range of possible emotions and feelings that cannot be readily discerned from the script of a play. The reader must add tone to the words to understand the full meaning of a passage. Recognizing tone is a cumulative process as the reader begins to understand the characters and situations in the play. Other elements that influence the interpretation of dialogue include the setting, possible reactions of the characters to the speech, and possible gestures or facial expressions of the actor. There are no firm rules to guide the interpretation of dramatic speech. An open and flexible attitude is essential in interpreting dramatic dialogue.

Action is a crucial element in the production of a dramatic work. Many dramas contain little dialogue and much action. In these cases, it is essential for the reader to carefully study stage directions and visualize the action on the stage. Benefits of understanding stage directions include knowing which characters are on the stage at all times, who is speaking to whom, and following these patterns through changes of scene.

Stage directions also provide additional information, some of which is not available to a live audience. The nature of the physical space where the action occurs is vital, and stage directions help with this. The historical context of the period is important in understanding what the playwright was working with in terms of theaters and physical space. The type of staging possible for the author is a good guide to the spatial elements of a production.

> ➤ **Review Video: Actions and Stage Directions**
> *Visit* **mometrix.com/academy** *and enter* **Code: 539974**

Asides and soliloquies are devices that authors use in plot and character development. **Asides** indicate that not all characters are privy to the lines. This may be a method of advancing or explaining the plot in a subtle manner. **Soliloquies** are opportunities for character development, plot enhancement, and to give insight to characters motives, feelings, and emotions. Careful study of these elements provides a reader with an abundance of clues to the major themes and plot of the work.

Art, music, and literature all interact in ways that contain many opportunities for the enrichment of all of the arts. Students could apply their knowledge of art and music by creating illustrations for a work or creating a musical score for a text. Students could discuss the meanings of texts and decide on their illustrations, or a score could amplify the meaning of the text.

Understanding the art and music of a period can make the experience of literature a richer, more rewarding experience. Students should be encouraged to use the knowledge of art and music to illuminate the text. Examining examples of dress, architecture, music, and dance of a period may be helpful in a fuller engagement of the text. Much of period literature lends itself to the analysis of the prevailing taste in art and music of an era, which helps place the literary work in a more meaningful context.

Testing tips

Skimming

Your first task when you begin reading is to answer the question "What is the topic of the selection?" This can best be answered by quickly skimming the passage for the general idea, stopping to read only the first sentence of each paragraph. A paragraph's first sentence is usually the main topic sentence, and it gives you a summary of the content of the paragraph.

Once you've skimmed the passage, stopping to read only the first sentences, you will have a general idea about what it is about, as well as what is the expected topic in each paragraph.

Each question will contain clues as to where to find the answer in the passage. Do not just randomly search through the passage for the correct answer to each question. Search scientifically. Find key word(s) or ideas in the question that are going to either contain or be near the correct answer. These are typically nouns, verbs, numbers, or phrases in the question that will probably be duplicated in the passage. Once you have identified those key word(s) or idea, skim the passage quickly to find where those key word(s) or idea appears. The correct answer choice will be nearby.

Example: What caused Martin to suddenly return to Paris?

The key word is Paris. Skim the passage quickly to find where this word appears. The answer will be close by that word.

However, sometimes key words in the question are not repeated in the passage. In those cases, search for the general idea of the question.

Example: Which of the following was the psychological impact of the author's childhood upon the remainder of his life?

- 30 -

Key words are "childhood" or "psychology". While searching for those words, be alert for other words or phrases that have similar meaning, such as "emotional effect" or "mentally" which could be used in the passage, rather than the exact word "psychology".

Numbers or years can be particularly good key words to skim for, as they stand out from the rest of the text.

Example: Which of the following best describes the influence of Monet's work in the 20th century?

20th contains numbers and will easily stand out from the rest of the text. Use 20th as the key word to skim for in the passage.

Other good key word(s) may be in quotation marks. These identify a word or phrase that is copied directly from the passage. In those cases, the word(s) in quotation marks are exactly duplicated in the passage.

Example: In her college years, what was meant by Margaret's "drive for excellence"?

"Drive for excellence" is a direct quote from the passage and should be easy to find.

Once you've quickly found the correct section of the passage to find the answer, focus upon the answer choices. Sometimes a choice will repeat word for word a portion of the passage near the answer. However, beware of such duplication – it may be a trap! More than likely, the correct choice will paraphrase or summarize the related portion of the passage, rather than being exactly the same wording.
For the answers that you think are correct, read them carefully and make sure that they answer the question. An answer can be factually correct, but it MUST answer the question asked. Additionally, two answers can both be seemingly correct, so be sure to read all of the answer choices, and make sure that you get the one that BEST answers the question.

Some questions will not have a key word.

Example: Which of the following would the author of this passage likely agree with?

In these cases, look for key words in the answer choices. Then skim the passage to find where the answer choice occurs. By skimming to find where to look, you can minimize the time required.

Sometimes it may be difficult to identify a good key word in the question to skim for in the passage. In those cases, look for a key word in one of the answer choices to skim for. Often the answer choices can all be found in the same paragraph, which can quickly narrow your search.

Paragraph Focus

Focus upon the first sentence of each paragraph, which is the most important. The main topic of the paragraph is usually there.

Once you've read the first sentence in the paragraph, you have a general idea about what each paragraph will be about. As you read the questions, try to determine which paragraph will have the answer. Paragraphs have a concise topic. The answer should either obviously be there or obviously not. It will save time if you can jump straight to the paragraph, so try to remember what you learned from the first sentences.
Example: The first paragraph is about poets; the second is about poetry. If a question asks about poetry, where will the answer be? The second paragraph.

The main idea of a passage is typically spread across all or most of its paragraphs. Whereas the main idea of a paragraph may be completely different than the main idea of the very next paragraph, a main idea for a passage affects all of the paragraphs in one form or another.
Example: What is the main idea of the passage?

For each answer choice, try to see how many paragraphs are related. It can help to count how many sentences are affected by each choice, but it is best to see how many paragraphs are affected by the choice. Typically the answer choices will include incorrect choices that are main ideas of individual paragraphs, but not the entire passage. That is why it is crucial to choose ideas that are supported by the most paragraphs possible.

Eliminate Choices

Some choices can quickly be eliminated. "Andy Warhol lived there." Is Andy Warhol even mentioned in the article? If not, quickly eliminate it.

When trying to answer a question such as "the passage indicates all of the following EXCEPT" quickly skim the paragraph searching for references to each choice. If the reference exists, scratch it off as a choice. Similar choices may be crossed off simultaneously if they are close enough.

In choices that ask you to choose "which answer choice does NOT describe?" or "all of the following answer choices are identifiable characteristics, EXCEPT which?" look for answers that are similarly worded. Since only one answer can be correct, if there are two answers that appear to mean the same thing, they must BOTH be incorrect, and can be eliminated.

Example:
A.)   changing values and attitudes
B.)   a large population of mobile or uprooted people

These answer choices are similar; they both describe a fluid culture. Because of their similarity, they can be linked together. Since the answer can have only one choice, they can also be eliminated together.

Contextual Clues

Look for contextual clues. An answer can be right but not correct. The contextual clues will help you find the answer that is most right and is correct. Understand the context in which a phrase is stated.

When asked for the implied meaning of a statement made in the passage, immediately go find the statement and read the context it was made in. Also, look for an answer choice that has a similar phrase to the statement in question.
Example: In the passage, what is implied by the phrase "Churches have become more or less part of the furniture"?

Find an answer choice that is similar or describes the phrase "part of the furniture" as that is the key phrase in the question. "Part of the furniture" is a saying that means something is fixed, immovable, or set in their ways. Those are all similar ways of saying "part of the furniture." As such, the correct answer choice will probably include a similar rewording of the expression.
Example: Why was John described as "morally desperate".

The answer will probably have some sort of definition of morals in it. "Morals" refers to a code of right and wrong behavior, so the correct answer choice will likely have words that mean something like that.

Fact/Opinion

When asked about which statement is a fact or opinion, remember that answer choices that are facts will typically have no ambiguous words. For example, how long is a long time? What defines an ordinary person? These ambiguous words of "long" and "ordinary" should not be in a factual statement. However, if all of the choices have ambiguous words, go to the context of the passage. Often a factual statement may be set out as a research finding.
Example: "The scientist found that the eye reacts quickly to change in light."

Opinions may be set out in the context of words like thought, believed, understood, or wished.
Example: "He thought the Yankees should win the World Series."

Opposites

Answer choices that are direct opposites are usually correct. The paragraph will often contain established relationships (when this goes up, that goes down). The

- 33 -

question may ask you to draw conclusions for this and will give two similar answer choices that are opposites.
Example:
A.) a decrease in housing starts
B.) an increase in housing starts

Make Predictions
As you read and understand the passage and then the question, try to guess what the answer will be. Remember that three of the four answer choices are wrong, and once you being reading them, your mind will immediately become cluttered with answer choices designed to throw you off. Your mind is typically the most focused immediately after you have read the passage and question and digested its contents. If you can, try to predict what the correct answer will be. You may be surprised at what you can predict.

Quickly scan the choices and see if your prediction is in the listed answer choices. If it is, then you can be quite confident that you have the right answer. It still won't hurt to check the other answer choices, but most of the time, you've got it!

Answer the Question
It may seem obvious to only pick answer choices that answer the question, but RN Pre-entrance exam can create some excellent answer choices that are wrong. Don't pick an answer just because it sounds right, or you believe it to be true. It MUST answer the question. Once you've made your selection, always go back and check it against the question and make sure that you didn't misread the question, and the answer choice does answer the question posed.

Benchmark
After you read the first answer choice, decide if you think it sounds correct or not. If it doesn't, move on to the next answer choice. If it does, make a mental note about that choice. This doesn't mean that you've definitely selected it as your answer choice, it just means that it's the best you've seen thus far. Go ahead and read the next choice. If the next choice is worse than the one you've already selected, keep going to the next answer choice. If the next choice is better than the choice you've already selected, then make a mental note about that answer choice.

As you read through the list, you are mentally noting the choice you think is right. That is your new standard. Every other answer choice must be benchmarked against that standard. That choice is correct until proven otherwise by another answer choice beating it out. Once you've decided that no other answer choice seems as good, do one final check to ensure that it answers the question posed.

New Information
Correct answers will usually contain the information listed in the paragraph and question. Rarely will completely new information be inserted into a correct answer

choice. Occasionally the new information may be related in a manner that RN Pre-entrance exam is asking for you to interpret, but seldom.

Example:

The argument above is dependent upon which of the following assumptions?

A.) Charles's Law was used

If Charles's Law is not mentioned at all in the referenced paragraph and argument, then it is unlikely that this choice is correct. All of the information needed to answer the question is provided for you, and so you should not have to make guesses that are unsupported or choose answer choices that have unknown information that cannot be reasoned.

Valid Information

Don't discount any of the information provided in the passage, particularly shorter ones. Every piece of information may be necessary to determine the correct answer. None of the information in the paragraph is there to throw you off (while the answer choices will certainly have information to throw you off). If two seemingly unrelated topics are discussed, don't ignore either. You can be confident there is a relationship, or it wouldn't be included in the paragraph, and you are probably going to have to determine what is that relationship for the answer.

Time Management

In technical passages, do not get lost on the technical terms. Skip them and move on. You want a general understanding of what is going on, not a mastery of the passage.

When you encounter material in the selection that seems difficult to understand, it often may not be necessary and can be skipped. Only spend time trying to understand it if it is going to be relevant for a question. Understand difficult phrases only as a last resort.

Answer general questions before detail questions. A reader with a good understanding of the whole passage can often answer general questions without rereading a word. Get the easier questions out of the way before tackling the more time consuming ones.

Identify each question by type. Usually the wording of a question will tell you whether you can find the answer by referring directly to the passage or by using your reasoning powers. You alone know which question types you customarily handle with ease and which give you trouble and will require more time. Save the difficult questions for last.

Final Warnings

Word Usage Questions

When asked how a word is used in the passage, don't use your existing knowledge of the word. The question is being asked precisely because there is some strange or unusual usage of the word in the passage. Go to the passage and use contextual clues to determine the answer. Don't simply use the popular definition you already know.

Switchback Words

Stay alert for "switchbacks". These are the words and phrases frequently used to alert you to shifts in thought. The most common switchback word is "but". Others include although, however, nevertheless, on the other hand, even though, while, in spite of, despite, regardless of.

Avoid "Fact Traps"

Once you know which paragraph the answer will be in, focus on that paragraph. However, don't get distracted by a choice that is factually true about the paragraph. Your search is for the answer that answers the question, which may be about a tiny aspect in the paragraph. Stay focused and don't fall for an answer that describes the larger picture of the paragraph. Always go back to the question and make sure you're choosing an answer that actually answers the question and is not just a true statement.

Mathematics Test Review

The Mathematics Test sections of the RN Pre-entrance exam consists of 40 questions.

Algebra

Numbers and their Classifications

Numbers are the basic building blocks of mathematics. Specific features of numbers are identified by the following terms:

Integers – The set of whole positive and negative numbers, including zero. Integers do not include fractions ($\frac{1}{3}$), decimals (0.56), or mixed numbers ($7\frac{3}{4}$).

Prime number – A whole number greater than 1 that has only two factors, itself and 1; that is, a number that can be divided evenly only by 1 and itself.

Composite number – A whole number greater than 1 that has more than two different factors; in other words, any whole number that is not a prime number. For example: The composite number 8 has the factors of 1, 2, 4, and 8.

Even number – Any integer that can be divided by 2 without leaving a remainder. For example: 2, 4, 6, 8, and so on.

Odd number – Any integer that cannot be divided evenly by 2. For example: 3, 5, 7, 9, and so on.

Decimal number – a number that uses a decimal point to show the part of the number that is less than one. Example: 1.234.

Decimal point – a symbol used to separate the ones place from the tenths place in decimals or dollars from cents in currency.

Decimal place – the position of a number to the right of the decimal point. In the decimal 0.123, the 1 is in the first place to the right of the decimal point, indicating tenths; the 2 is in the second place, indicating hundredths; and the 3 is in the third place, indicating thousandths.

The decimal, or base 10, system is a number system that uses ten different digits (0, 1, 2, 3, 4, 5, 6, 7, 8, 9). An example of a number system that uses something other than ten digits is the binary, or base 2, number system, used by computers, which uses only the numbers 0 and 1. It is thought that the decimal system originated because people had only their 10 fingers for counting.

Rational, irrational, and real numbers can be described as follows:
Rational numbers include all integers, decimals, and fractions. Any terminating or repeating decimal number is a rational number.
Irrational numbers cannot be written as fractions or decimals because the number of decimal places is infinite and there is no recurring pattern of digits within the number. For example, pi (π) begins with 3.141592 and continues without terminating or repeating, so pi is an irrational number.
Real numbers are the set of all rational and irrational numbers.

Operations

There are four basic mathematical operations:

Addition increases the value of one quantity by the value of another quantity. Example: $2 + 4 = 6; 8 + 9 = 17$. The result is called the sum. With addition, the order does not matter. $4 + 2 = 2 + 4$.

Subtraction is the opposite operation to addition; it decreases the value of one quantity by the value of another quantity. Example: $6 - 4 = 2; 17 - 8 = 9$. The result is called the difference. Note that with subtraction, the order does matter. $6 - 4 \neq 4 - 6$.

Multiplication can be thought of as repeated addition. One number tells how many times to add the other number to itself. Example: 3×2 (three times two) $= 2 + 2 + 2 = 6$. With multiplication, the order does not matter. $2 \times 3 = 3 \times 2$ or $3 + 3 = 2 + 2 + 2$.

Division is the opposite operation to multiplication; one number tells us how many parts to divide the other number into. Example: $20 \div 4 = 5$; if 20 is split into 4 equal parts, each part is 5. With division, the order of the numbers does matter. $20 \div 4 \neq 4 \div 20$.

An exponent is a superscript number placed next to another number at the top right. It indicates how many times the base number is to be multiplied by itself. Exponents provide a shorthand way to write what would be a longer mathematical expression. Example: $a^2 = a \times a; 2^4 = 2 \times 2 \times 2 \times 2$. A number with an exponent of 2 is said to be "squared," while a number with an exponent of 3 is said to be "cubed." The value of a number raised to an exponent is called its power. So, 8^4 is read as "8 to the 4th power," or "8 raised to the power of 4." A negative exponent is the same as the reciprocal of a positive exponent. Example: $a^{-2} = \frac{1}{a^2}$.

Parentheses are used to designate which operations should be done first when there are multiple operations. Example: 4 – (2 + 1) = 1; the parentheses tell us that we must add 2 and 1, and then subtract the sum from 4, rather than subtracting 2 from 4 and then adding 1 (this would give us an answer of 3).

Order of Operations is a set of rules that dictates the order in which we must perform each operation in an expression so that we will evaluate at accurately. If we have an expression that includes multiple different operations, Order of Operations tells us which operations to do first. The most common mnemonic for Order of Operations is PEMDAS, or "Please Excuse My Dear Aunt Sally." PEMDAS stands for Parentheses, Exponents, Multiplication, Division, Addition, Subtraction. It is important to understand that multiplication and division have equal precedence, as do addition and subtraction, so those pairs of operations are simply worked from left to right in order.

Example: Evaluate the expression $5 + 20 \div 4 \times (2 + 3)^2 - 6$ using the correct order of operations.

P: Perform the operations inside the parentheses, $(2 + 3) = 5$.

E: Simplify the exponents, $(5)^2 = 25$.

The equation now looks like this: $5 + 20 \div 4 \times 25 - 6$.

MD: Perform multiplication and division from left to right, $20 \div 4 = 5$; then $5 \times 25 = 125$.

The equation now looks like this: $5 + 125 - 6$.

AS: Perform addition and subtraction from left to right, $5 + 125 = 130$; then $130 - 6 = 124$.

The laws of exponents are as follows:

1)   Any number to the power of 1 is equal to itself: $a^1 = a$.

2)   The number 1 raised to any power is equal to 1: $1^n = 1$.

3)   Any number raised to the power of 0 is equal to 1: $a^0 = 1$.

4)   Add exponents to multiply powers of the same base number:$a^n \times a^m = a^{n+m}$.

5)   Subtract exponents to divide powers of the same number; that is $a^n \div a^m = a^{n-m}$.

6)   Multiply exponents to raise a power to a power: $(a^n)^m = a^{n \times m}$.

7)   If multiplied or divided numbers inside parentheses are collectively raised to a power, this is the same as each individual term being raised to that power: $(a \times b)^n = a^n \times b^n$; $(a \div b)^n = a^n \div b^n$.

Note: Exponents do not have to be integers. Fractional or decimal exponents follow all the rules above as well. Example: $5^{\frac{1}{4}} \times 5^{\frac{3}{4}} = 5^{\frac{1}{4}+\frac{3}{4}} = 5^1 = 5$.

> **Review Video: <u>Order of Operations</u>**
*Visit **mometrix.com/academy** and enter **Code: 259675***

A root, such as a square root, is another way of writing a fractional exponent. Instead of using a superscript, roots use the radical symbol ($\sqrt{}$) to indicate the operation. A radical will have a number underneath the bar, and may sometimes have a number in the upper left: $\sqrt[n]{a}$, read as "the nth root of a." The relationship between radical notation and exponent notation can be described by this equation: $\sqrt[n]{a} = a^{\frac{1}{n}}$. The two special cases of $n = 2$ and $n = 3$ are called square roots and cube roots. If there is no number to the upper left, it is understood to be a square root ($n = 2$). Nearly all of the roots you encounter will be square roots. A square root is the same as a number raised to the one-half power. When we say that a is the square root of b ($a = \sqrt{b}$), we mean that a multiplied by itself equals b: ($a \times a = b$).

A perfect square is a number that has an integer for its square root. There are 10 perfect squares from 1 to 100: 1, 4, 9, 16, 25, 36, 49, 64, 81, 100 (the squares of integers 1 through 10).

Scientific notation is a way of writing large numbers in a shorter form. The form $a \times 10^n$ is used in scientific notation, where a is greater than or equal to 1, but less than 10, and n is the number of places the decimal must move to get from the original number to a. Example: The number 230,400,000 is cumbersome to write. To write the value in scientific notation, place a decimal point between the first and second numbers, and include all digits through the last non-zero digit ($a = 2.304$). To find the appropriate power of 10, count the number of places the decimal point had to move ($n = 8$). The number is positive if the decimal moved to the left, and negative if it moved to the right. We can then write 230,400,000 as 2.304×10^8. If we look instead at the number 0.00002304, we have the same value for a, but this time the decimal moved 5 places to the right ($n = -5$). Thus, 0.00002304 can be written as 2.304×10^{-5}. Using this notation makes it simple to compare very large or very small numbers. By comparing exponents, it is easy to see that 3.28×10^4 is smaller than 1.51×10^5, because 4 is less than 5.

Positive & Negative Numbers
A precursor to working with negative numbers is understanding what absolute values are. A number's *Absolute Value* is simply the distance away from zero a number is on the number line. The absolute value of a number is always positive and is written $|x|$.

When adding signed numbers, if the signs are the same simply add the absolute values of the addends and apply the original sign to the sum. For example, $(+4) + (+8) = +12$ and $(-4) + (-8) = -12$. When the original signs are different, take the absolute values of the addends and subtract the smaller value from the larger value, then apply the original sign of the larger value to the difference. For instance, $(+4) + (-8) = -4$ and $(-4) + (+8) = +4$.

For subtracting signed numbers, change the sign of the number after the minus symbol and then follow the same rules used for addition. For example, $(+4) - (+8) = (+4) + (-8) = -4$.

> ➤ **Review Video: <u>Addition and Subtraction</u>**
> *Visit **mometrix.com/academy** and enter **Code: 521157***

If the signs are the same the product is positive when multiplying signed numbers. For example, $(+4) \times (+8) = +32$ and $(-4) \times (-8) = +32$. If the signs are opposite, the product is negative. For example, $(+4) \times (-8) = -32$ and $(-4) \times (+8) = -32$. When more than two factors are multiplied together, the sign of the product is determined by how many negative factors are present. If there are an odd number of negative factors then the product is negative, whereas an even number of negative factors indicates a positive product. For instance, $(+4) \times (-8) \times (-2) = +64$ and $(-4) \times (-8) \times (-2) = -64$.

The rules for dividing signed numbers are similar to multiplying signed numbers. If the dividend and divisor have the same sign, the quotient is positive. If the dividend and divisor have opposite signs, the quotient is negative. For example, $(-4) \div (+8) = -0.5$.

> ➤ **Review Video: <u>Multiplication and Division</u>**
> *Visit **mometrix.com/academy** and enter **Code: 643326***

Factors and Multiples

Factors are numbers that are multiplied together to obtain a product. For example, in the equation $2 \times 3 = 6$, the numbers 2 and 3 are factors. A prime number has only two factors (1 and itself), but other numbers can have many factors.

A common factor is a number that divides exactly into two or more other numbers. For example, the factors of 12 are 1, 2, 3, 4, 6, and 12, while the factors of 15 are 1, 3, 5, and 15. The common factors of 12 and 15 are 1 and 3.

A prime factor is also a prime number. Therefore, the prime factors of 12 are 2 and 3. For 15, the prime factors are 3 and 5.

The greatest common factor (GCF) is the largest number that is a factor of two or more numbers. For example, the factors of 15 are 1, 3, 5, and 15; the factors of 35 are 1, 5, 7, and 35. Therefore, the greatest common factor of 15 and 35 is 5.

The least common multiple (LCM) is the smallest number that is a multiple of two or more numbers. For example, the multiples of 3 include 3, 6, 9, 12, 15, etc.; the multiples of 5 include 5, 10, 15, 20, etc. Therefore, the least common multiple of 3 and 5 is 15.

> ➤ **Review Video: <u>Factors</u>**
> *Visit **mometrix.com/academy** and enter **Code: 920086***

Fractions, Percentages, and Related Concepts

A fraction is a number that is expressed as one integer written above another integer, with a dividing line between them $\left(\frac{x}{y}\right)$. It represents the quotient of the two numbers "x divided by y." It can also be thought of as x out of y equal parts.

The top number of a fraction is called the numerator, and it represents the number of parts under consideration. The 1 in $\frac{1}{4}$ means that 1 part out of the whole is being considered in the calculation. The bottom number of a fraction is called the denominator, and it represents the total number of equal parts. The 4 in $\frac{1}{4}$ means that the whole consists of 4 equal parts. A fraction cannot have a denominator of zero; this is referred to as "undefined."

Fractions can be manipulated, without changing the value of the fraction, by multiplying or dividing (but not adding or subtracting) both the numerator and denominator by the same number. If you divide both numbers by a common factor, you are reducing or simplifying the fraction. Two fractions that have the same value, but are expressed differently are known as equivalent fractions.

For example, $\frac{2}{10}, \frac{3}{15}, \frac{4}{20}$, and $\frac{5}{25}$ are all equivalent fractions. They can also all be reduced or simplified to $\frac{1}{5}$.

When two fractions are manipulated so that they have the same denominator, this is known as finding a common denominator. The number chosen to be that common denominator should be the least common multiple of the two original denominators. Example: $\frac{3}{4}$ and $\frac{5}{6}$; the least common multiple of 4 and 6 is 12. Manipulating to achieve the common denominator: $\frac{3}{4} = \frac{9}{12}; \frac{5}{6} = \frac{10}{12}$.

If two fractions have a common denominator, they can be added or subtracted simply by adding or subtracting the two numerators and retaining the same denominator. Example: $\frac{1}{2} + \frac{1}{4} = \frac{2}{4} + \frac{1}{4} = \frac{3}{4}$. If the two fractions do not already have the same denominator, one or both of them must be manipulated to achieve a common denominator before they can be added or subtracted.

Two fractions can be multiplied by multiplying the two numerators to find the new numerator and the two denominators to find the new denominator. Example: $\frac{1}{3} \times \frac{2}{3} = \frac{1 \times 2}{3 \times 3} = \frac{2}{9}$.
Two fractions can be divided flipping the numerator and denominator of the second fraction and then proceeding as though it were a multiplication. Example: $\frac{2}{3} \div \frac{3}{4} = \frac{2}{3} \times \frac{4}{3} = \frac{8}{9}$.

A fraction whose denominator is greater than its numerator is known as a proper fraction, while a fraction whose numerator is greater than its denominator is known as an improper fraction. Proper fractions have values less than one and improper fractions have values greater than one.

A mixed number is a number that contains both an integer and a fraction. Any improper fraction can be rewritten as a mixed number. Example: $\frac{8}{3} = \frac{6}{3} + \frac{2}{3} = 2 + \frac{2}{3} = 2\frac{2}{3}$. Similarly, any mixed number can be rewritten as an improper fraction. Example: $1\frac{3}{5} = 1 + \frac{3}{5} = \frac{5}{5} + \frac{3}{5} = \frac{8}{5}$.

> **Review Video: <u>Fractions</u>**
*Visit **mometrix.com/academy** and enter **Code: 262335***

Percentages can be thought of as fractions that are based on a whole of 100; that is, one whole is equal to 100%. The word percent means "per hundred." Fractions can be expressed as percents by finding equivalent fractions with a denomination of 100. Example: $\frac{7}{10} = \frac{70}{100} = 70\%; \frac{1}{4} = \frac{25}{100} = 25\%$.

To express a percentage as a fraction, divide the percentage number by 100 and reduce the fraction to its simplest possible terms. Example: $60\% = \frac{60}{100} = \frac{3}{5}$; $96\% = \frac{96}{100} = \frac{24}{25}$.

Converting decimals to percentages and percentages to decimals is as simple as moving the decimal point. To convert from a decimal to a percent, move the decimal point two places to the right. To convert from a percent to a decimal, move it two places to the left. Example: 0.23 = 23%; 5.34 = 534%; 0.007 = 0.7%; 700% = 7.00; 86% = 0.86; 0.15% = 0.0015.

It may be helpful to remember that the percentage number will always be larger than the equivalent decimal number.

A percentage problem can be presented three main ways: (1) Find what percentage of some number another number is. Example: What percentage of 40 is 8? (2) Find what number is some percentage of a given number. Example: What number is 20% of 40? (3) Find what number another number is a given percentage of. Example: What number is 8 20% of? The three components in all of these cases are the same: a whole (W), a part (P), and a percentage (%). These are related by the equation: $P = W \times \%$. This is the form of the equation you would use to solve problems of type (2). To solve types (1) and (3), you would use these two forms: $\% = \frac{P}{W}$ and $W = \frac{P}{\%}$.

The thing that frequently makes percentage problems difficult is that they are most often also word problems, so a large part of solving them is figuring out which quantities are what. Example: In a school cafeteria, 7 students choose pizza, 9 choose hamburgers, and 4 choose tacos. Find the percentage that chooses tacos. To find the whole, you must first add all of the parts: 7 + 9 + 4 = 20. The percentage can then be found by dividing the part by the whole ($\% = \frac{P}{W}$): $\frac{4}{20} = \frac{20}{100} = 20\%$.

A ratio is a comparison of two quantities in a particular order. Example: If there are 14 computers in a lab, and the class has 20 students, there is a student to computer ratio of 20 to 14, commonly written as 20:14. Ratios are normally reduced to their smallest whole number representation, so 20:14 would be reduced to 10:7 by dividing both sides by 2.

A proportion is a relationship between two quantities that dictates how one changes when the other changes. A direct proportion describes a relationship in which a quantity increases by a set amount for every increase in the other quantity, or decreases by that same amount for every decrease in the other quantity. Example: Assuming a constant driving speed, the time required for a car trip increases as the distance of the trip increases. The distance to be traveled and the time required to travel are directly proportional.

Inverse proportion is a relationship in which an increase in one quantity is accompanied by a decrease in the other, or vice versa. Example: the time required for a car trip decreases as the speed increases, and increases as the speed decreases, so the time required is inversely proportional to the speed of the car.

Equations and Graphing

When algebraic functions and equations are shown graphically, they are usually shown on a *Cartesian Coordinate Plane*. The Cartesian coordinate plane consists of two number lines placed perpendicular to each other, and intersecting at the zero point, also known as the origin. The horizontal number line is known as the *x*-axis, with positive values to the right of the origin, and negative values to the left of the origin. The vertical number line is known as the *y*-axis, with positive values above the origin, and negative values below the origin. Any point on the plane can be identified by an ordered pair in the form (*x,y*), called coordinates. The *x*-value of the coordinate is called the abscissa, and the *y*-value of the coordinate is called the ordinate. The two number lines divide the plane into four quadrants: I, II, III, and IV.

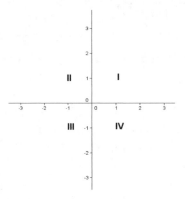

Before learning the different forms equations can be written in, it is important to understand some terminology. A ratio of the change in the vertical distance to the change in horizontal distance is called the *Slope*. On a graph with two points, (x_1, y_1) and (x_2, y_2), the slope is represented by the formula $= \frac{y_2 - y_1}{x_2 - x_1}$; $x_1 \neq x_2$. If the value of the slope is positive, the line slopes upward from left to right. If the value of the slope is negative, the line slopes downward from left to right. If the *y*-coordinates are the same for both points, the slope is 0 and the line is a *Horizontal Line*. If the *x*-coordinates are the same for both points, there is no slope and the line is a *Vertical Line*. Two or more lines that have equal slopes are *Parallel Lines. Perpendicular Lines* have slopes that are negative reciprocals of each other, such as $\frac{a}{b}$ and $\frac{-b}{a}$.

Equations are made up of monomials and polynomials. A *Monomial* is a single variable or product of constants and variables, such as x, $2x$, or $\frac{2}{x}$. There will never be addition or subtraction symbols in a monomial. Like monomials have like variables, but they may have different coefficients. *Polynomials* are algebraic expressions which use addition and subtraction to combine two or more

- 44 -

monomials. Two terms make a binomial; three terms make a trinomial; etc.. The *Degree of a Monomial* is the sum of the exponents of the variables. The *Degree of a Polynomial* is the highest degree of any individual term.

As mentioned previously, equations can be written many ways. Below is a list of the many forms equations can take.

- *Standard Form*: $Ax + By = C$; the slope is $\frac{-A}{B}$ and the y-intercept is $\frac{C}{B}$
- *Slope Intercept Form*: $y = mx + b$, where m is the slope and b is the y-intercept
- *Point-Slope Form*: $y - y_1 = m(x - x_1)$, where m is the slope and (x_1, y_1) is a point on the line
- *Two-Point Form*: $\frac{y-y_1}{x-x_1} = \frac{y_2-y_1}{x_2-x_1}$, where (x_1, y_1) and (x_2, y_2) are two points on the given line
- *Intercept Form*: $\frac{x}{x_1} + \frac{y}{y_1} = 1$, where $(x_1, 0)$ is the point at which a line intersects the x-axis, and $(0, y_1)$ is the point at which the same line intersects the y-axis

Equations can also be written as $ax + b = 0$, where $a \neq 0$. These are referred to as *One Variable Linear Equations*. A solution to such an equation is called a *Root*. In the case where we have the equation $5x + 10 = 0$, if we solve for x we get a solution of $x = -2$. In other words, the root of the equation is -2. This is found by first subtracting 10 from both sides, which gives $5x = -10$. Next, simply divide both sides by the coefficient of the variable, in this case 5, to get $x = -2$. This can be checked by plugging -2 back into the original equation $(5)(-2) + 10 = -10 + 10 = 0$.

The *Solution Set* is the set of all solutions of an equation. In our example, the solution set would simply be -2. If there were more solutions (there usually are in multivariable equations) then they would also be included in the solution set. When an equation has no true solutions, this is referred to as an *Empty Set*. Equations with identical solution sets are *Equivalent Equations*. An *Identity* is a term whose value or determinant is equal to 1.

Other Important Concepts
Commonly in algebra and other upper-level fields of math you find yourself working with mathematical expressions that do not equal each other. The statement comparing such expressions with symbols such as < (less than) or > (greater than) is called an *Inequality*. An example of an inequality is $7x > 5$. To solve for x, simply divide both sides by 7 and the solution is shown to be $x > \frac{5}{7}$. Graphs of the solution set of inequalities are represented on a number line. Open circles are used to show that an expression approaches a number but is never quite equal to that number.

Conditional Inequalities are those with certain values for the variable that will make the condition true and other values for the variable where the condition will be false. *Absolute Inequalities* can have any real number as the value for the variable to make the condition true, while there is no real number value for the variable that will make the condition false. Solving inequalities is done by following the same rules as for solving equations with the exception that when multiplying or dividing by a negative number the direction of the inequality sign must be flipped or reversed. *Double Inequalities* are situations where two inequality statements apply to the same variable expression. An example of this is $-c < ax + b < c$.

A *Weighted Mean*, or weighted average, is a mean that uses "weighted" values. The formula is weighted mean $= \frac{w_1 x_1 + w_2 x_2 + w_3 x_3 \ldots + w_n x_n}{w_1 + w_2 + w_3 + \cdots + w_n}$. Weighted values, such as $w_1, w_2, w_3, \ldots w_n$ are assigned to each member of the set $x_1, x_2, x_3, \ldots x_n$. If calculating weighted mean, make sure a weight value for each member of the set is used.

Calculations Using Points
Sometimes you need to perform calculations using only points on a graph as input data. Using points, you can determine what the midpoint and distance are. If you know the equation for a line you can calculate the distance between the line and the point.

To find the *Midpoint* of two points (x_1, y_1) and (x_2, y_2), average the x-coordinates to get the x-coordinate of the midpoint, and average the y-coordinates to get the y-coordinate of the midpoint. The formula is midpoint $= \left(\frac{x_1 + x_2}{2}, \frac{y_1 + y_2}{2} \right)$.

The *Distance* between two points is the same as the length of the hypotenuse of a right triangle with the two given points as endpoints, and the two sides of the right triangle parallel to the x-axis and y-axis, respectively. The length of the segment parallel to the x-axis is the difference between the x-coordinates of the two points. The length of the segment parallel to the y-axis is the difference between the y-coordinates of the two points. Use the Pythagorean Theorem $a^2 + b^2 = c^2$ or $c = \sqrt{a^2 + b^2}$ to find the distance. The formula is:
distance $= \sqrt{(x_2 - x_1)^2 + (y_2 - y_1)^2}$.

When a line is in the format $Ax + By + C = 0$, where A, B, and C are coefficients, you can use a point (x_1, y_1) not on the line and apply the formula $d = \frac{|Ax_1 + By_1 + C|}{\sqrt{A^2 + B^2}}$ to find the distance between the line and the point (x_1, y_1).

Systems of Equations
Systems of Equations are a set of simultaneous equations that all use the same variables. A solution to a system of equations must be true for each equation in the system. *Consistent Systems* are those with at least one solution. *Inconsistent Systems* are systems of equations that have no solution.

To solve a system of linear equations by *substitution*, start with the easier equation and solve for one of the variables. Express this variable in terms of the other variable. Substitute this expression in the other equation, and solve for the other variable. The solution should be expressed in the form (x, y). Substitute the values into both of the original equations to check your answer. Consider the following problem.

Solve the system using substitution:
$$x + 6y = 15$$
$$3x - 12y = 18$$
Solve the first equation for x:
$$x = 15 - 6y$$

Substitute this value in place of x in the second equation, and solve for y:
$$3(15 - 6y) - 12y = 18$$
$$45 - 18y - 12y = 18$$
$$30y = 27$$
$$y = \frac{27}{30} = \frac{9}{10} = 0.9$$
Plug this value for y back into the first equation to solve for x:
$$x = 15 - 6(0.9) = 15 - 5.4 = 9.6$$
Check both equations if you have time:
$$9.6 + 6(0.9) = 9.6 + 5.4 = 15$$
$$3(9.6) - 12(0.9) = 28.8 - 10.8 = 18$$
Therefore, the solution is $(9.6, 0.9)$.

To solve a system of equations using *elimination*, begin by rewriting both equations in standard form $Ax + By = C$. Check to see if the coefficients of one pair of like variables add to zero. If not, multiply one or both of the equations by a non-zero number to make one set of like variables add to zero. Add the two equations to solve for one of the variables. Substitute this value into one of the original equations to solve for the other variable. Check your work by substituting into the other equation. Next we will solve the same problem as above, but using the addition method.

Solve the system using elimination:
$$x + 6y = 15$$
$$3x - 12y = 18$$
If we multiply the first equation by 2, we can eliminate the y terms:
$$2x + 12y = 30$$
$$3x - 12y = 18$$

Add the equations together and solve for x:
$$5x = 48$$

$$x = \frac{48}{5} = 9.6$$

Plug the value for x back into either of the original equations and solve for y:
$$9.6 + 6y = 15$$
$$y = \frac{15 - 9.6}{6} = 0.9$$

Check both equations if you have time:
$$9.6 + 6(0.9) = 9.6 + 5.4 = 15$$
$$3(9.6) - 12(0.9) = 28.8 - 10.8 = 18$$

Therefore, the solution is (9.6, 0.9).

Polynomial Algebra

To multiply two binomials, follow the *FOIL* method. FOIL stands for:

- First: Multiply the first term of each binomial
- Outer: Multiply the outer terms of each binomial
- Inner: Multiply the inner terms of each binomial
- Last: Multiply the last term of each binomial

Using FOIL, $(Ax + By)(Cx + Dy) = ACx^2 + ADxy + BCxy + BDy^2$.

To divide polynomials, begin by arranging the terms of each polynomial in order of one variable. You may arrange in ascending or descending order, but be consistent with both polynomials. To get the first term of the quotient, divide the first term of the dividend by the first term of the divisor. Multiply the first term of the quotient by the entire divisor and subtract that product from the dividend. Repeat for the second and successive terms until you either get a remainder of zero or a remainder whose degree is less than the degree of the divisor. If the quotient has a remainder, write the answer as a mixed expression in the form: quotient $+ \frac{\text{remainder}}{\text{divisor}}$.

Rational Expressions are fractions with polynomials in both the numerator and the denominator; the value of the polynomial in the denominator cannot be equal to zero. To add or subtract rational expressions, first find the common denominator, then rewrite each fraction as an equivalent fraction with the common denominator. Finally, add or subtract the numerators to get the numerator of the answer, and keep the common denominator as the denominator of the answer. When multiplying rational expressions factor each polynomial and cancel like factors (a factor which appears in both the numerator and the denominator). Then, multiply all remaining factors in the numerator to get the numerator of the product, and multiply the remaining factors in the denominator to get the denominator of the product. Remember – cancel entire factors, not individual terms. To divide rational expressions, take the reciprocal of the divisor (the rational expression you are dividing by) and multiply by the dividend.

Below are patterns of some special products to remember: *perfect trinomial squares*, the *difference between two squares*, the *sum and difference of two cubes*, and *perfect cubes*.

- Perfect Trinomial Squares: $x^2 + 2xy + y^2 = (x + y)^2$ or $x^2 - 2xy + y^2 = (x - y)^2$
- Difference Between Two Squares: $x^2 - y^2 = (x + y)(x - y)$
- Sum of Two Cubes: $x^3 + y^3 = (x + y)(x^2 - xy + y^2)$
  Note: the second factor is NOT the same as a perfect trinomial square, so do not try to factor it further.
- Difference Between Two Cubes: $x^3 - y^3 = (x - y)(x^2 + xy + y^2)$
  Again, the second factor is NOT the same as a perfect trinomial square.
- Perfect Cubes: $x^3 + 3x^2y + 3xy^2 + y^3 = (x + y)^3$ and $x^3 - 3x^2y + 3xy^2 - y^3 = (x - y)^3$

In order to *factor* a polynomial, first check for a common monomial factor. When the greatest common monomial factor has been factored out, look for patterns of special products: differences of two squares, the sum or difference of two cubes for binomial factors, or perfect trinomial squares for trinomial factors. If the factor is a trinomial but not a perfect trinomial square, look for a factorable form, such as $x^2 + (a + b)x + ab = (x + a)(x + b)$ or $(ac)x^2 + (ad + bc)x + bd = (ax + b)(cx + d)$. For factors with four terms, look for groups to factor. Once you have found the factors, write the original polynomial as the product of all the factors. Make sure all of the polynomial factors are prime. Monomial factors may be prime or composite. Check your work by multiplying the factors to make sure you get the original polynomial.

Solving Quadratic Equations
The *Quadratic Formula* is used to solve quadratic equations when other methods are more difficult. To use the quadratic formula to solve a quadratic equation, begin by rewriting the equation in standard form $ax^2 + bx + c = 0$, where a, b, and c are coefficients. Once you have identified the values of the coefficients, substitute those values into the quadratic formula $x = \frac{-b \pm \sqrt{b^2 - 4ac}}{2a}$. Evaluate the equation and simplify the expression. Again, check each root by substituting into the original equation. In the quadratic formula, the portion of the formula under the radical $(b^2 - 4ac)$ is called the *Discriminant*. If the discriminant is zero, there is only one root: zero. If the discriminant is positive, there are two different real roots. If the discriminant is negative, there are no real roots.

To solve a quadratic equation by *Factoring*, begin by rewriting the equation in standard form, if necessary. Factor the side with the variable then set each of the factors equal to zero and solve the resulting linear equations. Check your answers by substituting the roots you found into the original equation. If, when writing the equation in standard form, you have an equation in the form $x^2 + c = 0$ or $x^2 - c = 0$, set $x^2 = -c$ or $x^2 = c$ and take the square root of c. If $c = 0$, the only real root is zero. If c is positive, there are two real roots—the positive and negative square root values. If c is negative, there are no real roots because you cannot take the square root of a negative number.

To solve a quadratic equation by *Completing the Square*, rewrite the equation so that all terms containing the variable are on the left side of the equal sign, and all the constants are on the right side of the equal sign. Make sure the coefficient of the squared term is 1. If there is a coefficient with the squared term, divide each term on both sides of the equal side by that number. Next, work with the coefficient of the single-variable term. Square half of this coefficient, and add that value to both sides. Now you can factor the left side (the side containing the variable) as the square of a binomial. $x^2 + 2ax + a^2 = C \Rightarrow (x + a)^2 = C$, where x is the variable, and a and C are constants. Take the square root of both sides and solve for the variable. Substitute the value of the variable in the original problem to check your work.

Geometry

Geometry concepts
Below are some terms that are commonly used in geometric studies. Most of these concepts are foundational to geometry, so understanding them is a necessary first step to studying geometry.

A point is a fixed location in space; has no size or dimensions; commonly represented by a dot.

A line is a set of points that extends infinitely in two opposite directions. It has length, but no width or depth. A line can be defined by any two distinct points that it contains. A line segment is a portion of a line that has definite endpoints. A ray is a portion of a line that extends from a single point on that line in one direction along the line. It has a definite beginning, but no ending.

A plane is a two-dimensional flat surface defined by three non-collinear points. A plane extends an infinite distance in all directions in those two dimensions. It contains an infinite number of points, parallel lines and segments, intersecting lines and segments, as well as parallel or intersecting rays. A plane will never contain a three-dimensional figure or skew lines. Two given planes will either be parallel or they will intersect to form a line. A plane may intersect a circular conic surface, such as a cone, to form conic sections, such as the parabola, hyperbola, circle or ellipse.

Perpendicular lines are lines that intersect at right angles. They are represented by the symbol ⊥. The shortest distance from a line to a point not on the line is a perpendicular segment from the point to the line.

Parallel lines are lines in the same plane that have no points in common and never meet. It is possible for lines to be in different planes, have no points in common, and never meet, but they are not parallel because they are in different planes.

A bisector is a line or line segment that divides another line segment into two equal lengths. A perpendicular bisector of a line segment is composed of points that are equidistant from the endpoints of the segment it is dividing.

Intersecting lines are lines that have exactly one point in common. Concurrent lines are multiple lines that intersect at a single point.

A transversal is a line that intersects at least two other lines, which may or may not be parallel to one another. A transversal that intersects parallel lines is a common occurrence in geometry.

➢ **Review Video: Geometry**
*Visit **mometrix.com/academy** and enter **Code: 425032***

Angles

An angle is formed when two lines or line segments meet at a common point. It may be a common starting point for a pair of segments or rays, or it may be the intersection of lines. Angles are represented by the symbol ∠.

The vertex is the point at which two segments or rays meet to form an angle. If the angle is formed by intersecting rays, lines, and/or line segments, the vertex is the point at which four angles are formed. The pairs of angles opposite one another are called vertical angles, and their measures are equal. In the figure below, angles ABC and DBE are congruent, as are angles ABD and CBE.

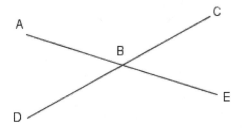

An acute angle is an angle with a degree measure less than 90°.
A right angle is an angle with a degree measure of exactly 90°.
An obtuse angle is an angle with a degree measure greater than 90° but less than 180°.

A straight angle is an angle with a degree measure of exactly 180°. This is also a semicircle.
A reflex angle is an angle with a degree measure greater than 180° but less than 360°.
A full angle is an angle with a degree measure of exactly 360°.

Two angles whose sum is exactly 90° are said to be complementary. The two angles may or may not be adjacent. In a right triangle, the two acute angles are complementary.

Two angles whose sum is exactly 180° are said to be supplementary. The two angles may or may not be adjacent. Two intersecting lines always form two pairs of supplementary angles. Adjacent supplementary angles will always form a straight line.

Two angles that have the same vertex and share a side are said to be adjacent. Vertical angles are not adjacent because they share a vertex but no common side.

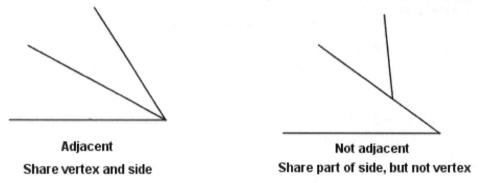

Adjacent
Share vertex and side

Not adjacent
Share part of side, but not vertex

When two parallel lines are cut by a transversal, the angles that are between the two parallel lines are interior angles. In the diagram below, angles 3, 4, 5, and 6 are interior angles.

When two parallel lines are cut by a transversal, the angles that are outside the parallel lines are exterior angles. In the diagram below, angles 1, 2, 7, and 8 are exterior angles.

When two parallel lines are cut by a transversal, the angles that are in the same position relative to the transversal and a parallel line are corresponding angles. The diagram below has four pairs of corresponding angles: angles 1 and 5; angles 2 and 6; angles 3 and 7; and angles 4 and 8. Corresponding angles formed by parallel lines are congruent.

When two parallel lines are cut by a transversal, the two interior angles that are on opposite sides of the transversal are called alternate interior angles. In the diagram below, there are two pairs of alternate interior angles: angles 3 and 6, and angles 4 and 5. Alternate interior angles formed by parallel lines are congruent.

When two parallel lines are cut by a transversal, the two exterior angles that are on opposite sides of the transversal are called alternate exterior angles. In the diagram below, there are two pairs of alternate exterior angles: angles 1 and 8, and angles 2 and 7. Alternate exterior angles formed by parallel lines are congruent.

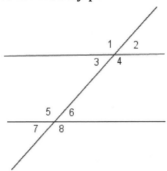

> ➢ **Review Video: Angles**
> *Visit **mometrix.com/academy** and enter **Code: 264624***

Circles
The center is the single point inside the circle that is equidistant from every point on the circle. (Point *O* in the diagram below.)

The radius is a line segment that joins the center of the circle and any one point on the circle. All radii of a circle are equal. (Segments *OX*, *OY*, and *OZ* in the diagram below.)

The diameter is a line segment that passes through the center of the circle and has both endpoints on the circle. The length of the diameter is exactly twice the length of the radius. (Segment *XZ* in the diagram below.)

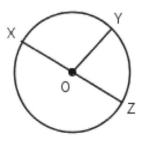

A circle is inscribed in a polygon if each of the sides of the polygon is tangent to the circle. A polygon is inscribed in a circle if each of the vertices of the polygon lies on the circle.

- 53 -

A circle is circumscribed about a polygon if each of the vertices of the polygon lies on the circle. A polygon is circumscribed about the circle if each of the sides of the polygon is tangent to the circle.

If one figure is inscribed in another, then the other figure is circumscribed about the first figure.

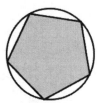

Circle circumscribed about a pentagon
Pentagon inscribed in a circle

Polygons
A polygon is a planar shape formed from line segments called sides that are joined together at points called vertices (singular: vertex). Specific polygons are named by the number of angles or sides they have. Regular polygons are polygons whose sides are all equal and whose angles are all congruent.

An interior angle is any of the angles inside a polygon where two sides meet at a vertex. The sum of the interior angles of a polygon is dependent only on the number of sides. For example, all 5-sided polygons have interior angles that sum to 540°, regardless of the particular shape.
A diagonal is a line that joins two nonconsecutive vertices of a polygon. The number of diagonals that can be drawn on an n-sided polygon is $d = \frac{n(n-3)}{2}$.

The following list presents several different types of polygons:
Triangle – 3 sides
Quadrilateral – 4 sides
Pentagon – 5 sides
Hexagon – 6 sides
Heptagon – 7 sides
Octagon – 8 sides
Nonagon – 9 sides
Decagon – 10 sides
Dodecagon – 12 sides

More generally, an n-gon is a polygon that has n angles and n sides.

The sum of the interior angles of an *n*-sided polygon is (n − 2)180°. For example, in a triangle n = 3, so the sum of the interior angles is (3 − 2)180° = 180°. In a quadrilateral, n = 4, and the sum of the angles is (4 − 2)180° = 360°. The sum of the interior angles of a polygon is equal to the sum of the interior angles of any other polygon with the same number of sides.

Below are descriptions for several common quadrilaterals. Recall that a quadrilateral is a four-sided polygon.

Trapezoid – quadrilateral with exactly one pair of parallel sides (opposite one another); in an isosceles trapezoid, the two non-parallel sides have equal length and both pairs of non-opposite angles are congruent
Parallelogram – quadrilateral with two pairs of parallel sides (opposite one another), and two pairs of congruent angles (opposite one another)
Rhombus – parallelogram with four equal sides
Rectangle – parallelogram with four congruent angles (right angles)
Square – parallelogram with four equal sides and four congruent angles (right angles)

Triangles
A triangle is a polygon with three sides and three angles. Triangles can be classified according to the length of their sides or magnitude of their angles.

An acute triangle is a triangle whose three angles are all less than 90°. If two of the angles are equal, the acute triangle is also an isosceles triangle. If the three angles are all equal, the acute triangle is also an equilateral triangle.

A right triangle is a triangle with exactly one angle equal to 90°. All right triangles follow the Pythagorean Theorem. A right triangle can never be acute or obtuse.

An obtuse triangle is a triangle with exactly one angle greater than 90°. The other two angles may or may not be equal. If the two remaining angles are equal, the obtuse triangle is also an isosceles triangle.

An equilateral triangle is a triangle with three congruent sides. An equilateral triangle will also have three congruent angles, each 60°. All equilateral triangles are also acute triangles.

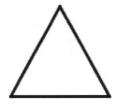

An isosceles triangle is a triangle with two congruent sides. An isosceles triangle will also have two congruent angles opposite the two congruent sides.

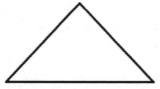

A scalene triangle is a triangle with no congruent sides. A scalene triangle will also have three angles of different measures. The angle with the largest measure is opposite the longest side, and the angle with the smallest measure is opposite the shortest side.

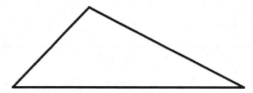

The Triangle Inequality Theorem states that the sum of the measures of any two sides of a triangle is always greater than the measure of the third side. If the sum of the measures of two sides were equal to the third side, a triangle would be impossible because the two sides would lie flat across the third side and there would be no vertex. If the sum of the measures of two of the sides was less than the third side, a closed figure would be impossible because the two shortest sides would never meet.

Similar triangles are triangles whose corresponding angles are congruent to one another. Their corresponding sides may or may not be equal, but they are proportional to one another. Since the angles in a triangle always sum to 180°, it is only necessary to determine that two pairs of corresponding angles are congruent, since the third will be also in that case.

Congruent triangles are similar triangles whose corresponding sides are all equal. Congruent triangles can be made to fit on top of one another by rotation, reflection, and/or translation. When trying to determine whether two triangles are congruent, there are several criteria that can be used.

Side-side-side (SSS): if all three sides of one triangle are equal to all three sides of another triangle, they are congruent by SSS.
Side-angle-side (SAS): if two sides and the adjoining angle in one triangle are equal to two sides and the adjoining angle of another triangle, they are congruent by SAS. Additionally, if two triangles can be shown to be similar, then there need only be one pair of corresponding equal sides to show congruence.

One of the most important theorems in geometry is the Pythagorean Theorem. Named after the sixth-century Greek mathematician Pythagoras, this theorem states that, for a right triangle, the square of the hypotenuse (the longest side of the triangle, always opposite the right angle) is equal to the sum of the squares of the other two sides. Written symbolically, the Pythagorean Theorem can be expressed as $a^2 + b^2 = c^2$, where c is the hypotenuse and a and b are the remaining two sides.

The theorem is most commonly used to find the length of an unknown side of a right triangle, given the lengths of the other two sides. For example, given that the hypotenuse of a right triangle is 5 and one side is 3, the other side can be found using the formula: $a^2 + b^2 = c^2, 3^2 + b^2 = 5^2, 9 + b^2 = 25, b^2 = 25 - 9 = 16,$ $b = \sqrt{16} = 4$.

The theorem can also be used "in reverse" to show that when the square of one side of a triangle is equal to the sum of the squares of the other two sides, the triangle must be a right triangle.

The Law of Sines states that $\frac{\sin A}{a} = \frac{\sin B}{b} = \frac{\sin C}{c}$, where A, B, and C are the angles of a triangle, and a, b, and c are the sides opposite their respective angles. This formula will work with all triangles, not just right triangles.

The Law of Cosines is given by the formula $c^2 = a^2 + b^2 - 2ab(\cos C)$, where a, b, and c are the sides of a triangle, and C is the angle opposite side c. This formula is similar to the Pythagorean Theorem, but unlike the Pythagorean Theorem, it can be used on any triangle.

Symmetry

Symmetry is a property of a shape in which the shape can be transformed by either reflection or rotation without losing its original shape and orientation. A shape that has reflection symmetry can be reflected across a line with the result being the same shape as before the reflection. A line of symmetry divides a shape into two parts, with each part being a mirror image of the other. A shape can have more than one line of symmetry. A circle, for instance, has an infinite number of lines of symmetry. When reflection symmetry is extended to three-dimensional space, it is taken to describe a solid that can be divided into mirror image parts by a plane of symmetry. Rotational symmetry describes a shape that can be rotated about a point and achieve its original shape and orientation with less than a 360° rotation. When rotational symmetry is extended to three-dimensional space, it describes a solid that can be rotated about a line with the same conditions. Many shapes have both reflection and rotational symmetry.

Area formulas

Rectangle: $A = wl$, where w is the width and l is the length

Square: $A = s^2$, where s is the length of a side.

Triangle: $A = \frac{1}{2}bh$, where b is the length of one side (base) and h is the distance from that side to the opposite vertex measured perpendicularly (height).

Parallelogram: $A = bh$, where b is the length of one side (base) and h is the perpendicular distance between that side and its parallel side (height).

Trapezoid: $A = \frac{1}{2}(b_1 + b_2)h$, where b_1 and b_2 are the lengths of the two parallel sides (bases), and h is the perpendicular distance between them (height).

Circle: $A = \pi r^2$, where π is the mathematical constant approximately equal to 3.14 and r is the distance from the center of the circle to any point on the circle (radius).

Volume Formulas

For some of these shapes, it is necessary to find the area of the base polygon before the volume of the solid can be found. This base area is represented in the volume equations as B.

Pyramid – consists of a polygon base, and triangles connecting each side of that polygon to a vertex. The volume can be calculated as $V = \frac{1}{3}Bh$, where h is the distance between the vertex and the base polygon, measured perpendicularly.

Prism – consists of two identical polygon bases, attached to one another on corresponding sides by parallelograms. The volume can be calculated as $V = Bh$, where h is the perpendicular distance between the two bases.

Cube – a special type of prism in which the two bases are the same shape as the side faces. All faces are squares. The volume can be calculated as $V = s^3$, where s is the length of any side.

Sphere – a round solid consisting of one continuous, uniformly-curved surface. The volume can be calculated as $V = \frac{4}{3}\pi r^3$, where r is the distance from the center of the sphere to any point on the surface (radius).

Science Test Review

The 60 minute Science Test consists of 60 questions. These questions will test your knowledge of basic principles and concepts in biology, chemistry, and physics.

While a general knowledge of these subjects is important, a complete mastery of them is NOT necessary to succeed on the Science Test. Don't be intimidated by the questions presented. They do not require highly advanced knowledge, but only the ability to recognize common problem types and apply basic principles and concepts to solving them.

That is our goal, to show you the simple methods to solving these problems, so that while you will not gain a mastery of these subjects from this guide, you will learn the methods necessary to succeed on the RN Pre-entrance exam.

This test may scare you. It may have been years since you've studied some of the basic concepts covered, and for even the most accomplished and studied student, these terms may be unfamiliar. General test-taking skill will help the most. DO NOT run out of time, move quickly, and use the easy pacing methods we outlined in the test-taking tactics section.

The most important thing you can do is to ignore your fears and jump into the test immediately- do not be overwhelmed by any strange-sounding terms. You have to jump into the test like jumping into a pool- all at once is the easiest way. Managing your time on this test can prove to be extremely difficult, as some of the questions may leave you stumped and countless minutes may waste away while you rack your brain for the answer. To be successful though, you must work efficiently and get through the entire test before running out of time.

Circulatory System

The cardiovascular system is vital for providing oxygen and nutrients to tissues and removing waste. The heart is divided into four chambers-two atria and two ventricles-that communicate through orifices on each side. The right atrium receives blood from the venous system and then lets blood fall down into the right ventricle. Blood then goes to the lungs for a new supply of oxygen. Then the blood comes back from the lungs and goes to the left atrium. It then falls into the left ventricle and is pumped into the general circulation. The heart is composed of three layers: epicardium, myocardium and an endocardium. Heart sounds are due to the vibrations produced by blood and valve movements. Blood pressure is the force exerted by blood against the insides of the blood vessels. Heart rate is determined by physical activity, body temperature, and concentration of ions. The heart is controlled by impulses from the S-A node which passes to the A-V node.

The arterial system is responsible for delivering oxygen to various tissues and the venous system is responsible for removing waste and returning blood to the heart.

Hypertension, is characterized by elevated arterial pressure and is one of the more common diseases of the cardiovascular system. Arteriosclerosis is accompanied by decreased elasticity of the arterial walls and followed by narrowing of the lumen. Hormones can also play a large role in blood pressure regulation. The hormone *aldosterone* can promote retention of water in the kidneys and increased blood volume, which in turn increases blood pressure.

Key Terms

Tachycardia-abnormally fast heartbeat
Bradycardia-abnormally slow heartbeat
Fibrillation-rapid heart beats
Red blood cell (erythrocyte)- transports carbon dioxide and oxygen
White blood cell (leukocyte)- fight infection including neutrophils, eosinophils, and basophils

Blood is made up of approximately 45% hematocrit, and 55% plasma. Plasma is primarily water, however contains approx. 7% protein and 1.5 other substances. The proteins found in plasma are: albumin, globulin and fibrinogen. Hematocrit is made up of mostly red blood cells, but also white blood cells and platelets. Platelets can be key in blood clotting to form a plug.

Respiratory Review

The respiratory stem includes the nose, nasal cavity, sinuses, pharynx, larynx, trachea, bronchial tree, and lungs. Air enters the nose, travels through the nasal cavity where the air is warmed. The air goes through the pharynx, which functions as a common duct for air and food. Then the larynx, which is at the top of the trachea and holds the vocal cords allows passage of air. The trachea divides into the right and left bronchi on the way into the bronchial tree and the lungs.

The right lung has three lobes and the left lung has two lobes. Gas exchange occurs between the air and the blood within the alveoli, which are tiny air sacs. Diffusion is the mechanism by which oxygen and carbon dioxide are exchanged.

Breathing is controlled by the medulla oblongata and pons. Inspiration is controlled by changes in the thoracic cavity. Air fills the lung because of atmospheric pressure pushing air in. Expansion of the lungs is aided by surface tension, which holds pleural membranes together. In addition, the diaphragm, which is located just below the lungs, and stimulated by phrenic nerve acts as a suction pump to encourage inspiration. Expiration comes from the recoil of tissues and the surface tension of the alveoli.

Aerobic respiration occurs in the presence of oxygen and mostly takes place in the mitochondria of a cell. Anaerobic respiration occurs in the absence of oxygen and takes place in the cytoplasm of a cell. Both of these mechanisms occur in cellular respiration in humans. With anaerobic respiration glucose is broken down and produces less ATP when compared to aerobic respiration.

Key Terms

Anoxia- absence of oxygen in tissue
Atelectasis- collapse of a lung
Dyspnea- difficulty in the breathing cycle
Hypercapnia- excessive carbon dioxide in the blood
Tidal Volume-amount of air that normally moves in and out of the lungs

Nervous System

The nervous system is made of the central nervous system (CNS) and the peripheral nervous system (PNS). The central nervous system is made up of the brain and the spinal cord. The peripheral nervous system consists of cranial and spinal nerves that innervate organs, muscles and sensory systems. The brain controls: thought, reasoning, memory, sight, and judgement. The brain is made up of four lobes: frontal, parietal, temporal, and occipital. The spinal cord is a made up of neural tracts that conduct information to and from the brain.

Cranial nerves in the peripheral nervous system connect the brain to the head, neck and trunk. Peripheral nerves allow control of muscle groups in the upper and lower extremities and sensory stimulation. The peripheral nerves are spinal nerves that branch off the spinal cord going toward organs, and muscles.

The autonomic nervous system controls reflexive functions of the brain. Including "fight or flight" response and maintaining homeostasis. Homeostasis is a state of equilibrium within tissues. The autonomic nervous system uses neurotransmitters to help conduct nerve signals and turn on/off various cell groups.

Nervous tissue is composed of neurons, which are the functional unit of the nervous system. A neuron includes a cell body, and organelles usually found in cells. Dendrites provide receptive information to the neuron and a single axon carries the information away.

> ➢ **Review Video: <u>Nervous System</u>**
> *Visit **mometrix.com/academy** and enter **Code: 708428***

Key Terms
Synapse- junction between two neurons
Action potential- threshold at which neurons fire

Digestive System

Digestion is a process that food is absorbed. The mouth begins to prepare food for digestion. Teeth grind food into smaller substrates. Then salivary glands, which secrete saliva, begin digestion of the food using enzymes. The pharynx and esophagus allow passage of the food into the stomach. The stomach uses gastric juices and absorbs a small amount of the food. Then, the food goes to the small intestine. The pancreas and the liver release enzymes and bile respectively into the small intestine to aid in absorption. The small intestine is composed of the duodenum, jejunum, and ileum. Then, substrates are passed into the large intestine, which has little digestive function. Absorption of water and electrolytes does occur in the large intestine.

Peristalsis is the wave like movement occurring in the digestive system that propels food downward. The alimentary canal is the path food travels from the mouth to the anus. Feces are composed mostly of water and substrates and are not absorbed.

Key Terms

Cholelithiasis- stones in the gallbladder
Diverticulitis- inflammation of the small pouches in the colon, if present
Hepatitis- inflammation of the liver
Stomatitis- inflammation of the mouth
Dyspepsia- indigestion
Enteritis- inflammation of the intestine

Reproductive System

Male reproductive organs are specialized for the formation of sperm (gamete) and transporting sperm. The vas deferens is the tube that sperm travels through. Semen is composed of sperm cells and secretions of the prostate and bulbourethral glands. Semen activates sperm cells.

Testosterone is the most important male hormone. Testosterone encourages the development of male sex organs. It is responsible for the development of male secondary sexual characteristics.

Female reproductive organs are specialized for childbirth and development of a fetus. The primary structures are the ovaries, uterus, and vagina. The ovaries release an egg cell (gamete) into the uterus. The uterus sustains life for the embryo until childbirth. The vagina allows transportation of the fetus during delivery.

Estrogen and progesterone are the primary female sex hormones. Estrogen is responsible for female sexual characteristics. Progesterone is responsible for changes in the uterus. Menopause is related to low estrogen levels and changes in the female reproductive organs. The product of fertilization is a zygote with 46 chromosomes.

Key Terms

Amenorrhea- absence of menstrual flow
Gestation- 40 weeks of pregnancy
Orchitis- inflammation of a testis
Cesarean section- birth of a fetus through an abdominal incision

Urinary System

The urinary system consists of the kidneys, ureters, bladder, and urethra. The kidney functions to remove metabolic wastes from the blood and excrete them. The also help regulate blood pressure, pH of the blood, and red blood cell production. The basic functional unit of the kidney is the nephron. The nephron consists of a renal corpuscle and a renal tubule. Urine is the end product of the urinary system. The kidneys are involved in filtration, re-absorption and secretion. Glomerular filtration is regulated by osmotic pressure.

The ureter is a tube that connects the kidneys and the bladder. Kidney stones can become lodged in the ureter. Peristaltic waves in the ureter force urine to the bladder. The bladder stores urine and forces urine into the urethra. Muscle fibers in the wall of the bladder form the detrusor muscle.

Key Terms

Enuresis-uncontrolled urination
Diuretic- a substance that encourages urination
Pyuria- pus in the urine
Ureteritis- inflammation of the ureter

Ear

The external ear collects sound and passes the sound to the tympanic membrane. Then the middle ear increases the force of the sound waves using the malleus, stapes, and incus. Auditory tubes connect the middle ear to throat and help maintain proper pressure. The inner ear consists of complex system of tubes and chambers-osseous, membranous labyrinths and also the cochlea. Auditory impulses are interpreted in the temporal lobes.

Eye

The wall of the eye has an outer, middle and inner layer. The sclera (outer layer) is protective. The cornea refracts light entering the eye and is found on the anterior aspect of the sclera. The choroid coat (middle layer) helps keep the inside of the eye dark. The retina (inner layer) contains the receptor cells. The visual receptors are rods and cones. Rods are responsible for colorless vision in dim light, and cones are responsible for color vision.

Key Terms

Otitis media- inflammation of the middle ear
Diplopia- double vision
Tinnitus- ringing in the ears
Vertigo-sensation of dizziness

Element Review

Fluorine, Chlorine, Bromide and Iodine are all halogens also known as salt formers. Helium, Neon, Argon, Krypton and Xenon are all inert gases also known as noble gases.
Lithium, Sodium, Potassium, Rubidium, and Cesium are all alkali metals.

The following periodic table presentation of Chlorine can be broken down into the following:

17	-	Atomic number
Cl	-	Element symbol
Chlorine	-	Element name
34.45	-	Atomic Weight

The horizontal rows of the periodic table are called periods. From left to right these are arranged by increasing atomic numbers. The vertical rows have similar chemical similarities. The number of known chemical elements is 109. The periodic table was created by, Dmitri Mendeleev a Russian chemist.

An atom is the simplest unit of an element. Atoms that loose or gain electrons are called ions. Positively charged ions are called cations. Negatively charged ions are called anions. All atoms have a nucleus, which has protons and neutrons present. Protons are positively charged particles found within the nucleus. Neutrons do not carry a charge. The total of neutrons and protons is the mass number. The atomic number is the number of protons found in an atom. One mole of that element is the weight of the element required to equal its atomic weight. A compound is when 2 elements are found together in a definite ratio. The term molecule is a unit of two or more atoms that are bonded together. Avogadro's number 6.02×10^{23} is the number of molecules in one mole of that element.

Atoms can share electrons to bond called a covalent bond, or they can transfer electrons to another atom to form an ionic bond. In addition, a polar bond may be performed between substances in situations that a covalent or ionic bond is not desired. Compounds with various structures, but the same shape are called isomers.

Substances can exist in various states of matter. The three common states of matter are solid, liquid, and gas. Water can exist in all three forms. At 0 degrees Celsius water is a solid. At 100 degrees Celsius water becomes a gas. In solid form the molecules of water are moving very slowly. In liquid form the molecules of water are moving at a faster pace, and in gas form are highly excited. Converting liquid into a gas is known as evaporation. Converting gas into a liquid is known as condensation. Due to the fact that liquids and gases flow easily they are known as fluids. Transfer of a solid into a gas without going through the liquid state is known as sublimation.

Energy taken in or given off during reactions is measured as heat. Heat can be measured in various units. Units include: joule-.239 calories, calorie-degree of energy required to raise one gram of water at 14.5 Celsius degrees by a single degree of Celsius.

Solutions

The concept of solvent and solute are applicable to gases, liquids and solids. A solvent is the host substance and the solute is the substance that is can be dissolved in the solvent. A solution is a mixture with same composition made of 2 or more substances. A solution that contains the maximum amount of solute is called a saturated solution. A heterogenous mixture is a solution that contains unequal distribution of solvents in the solution. A physical change is a change in the state of matter. A chemical change is a change in the chemical composition of a compound.

When discussing acid and base relationships. An acid is substance that increases the hydrogen ion concentration in water. A base is a substance that increases the hydroxide ion count in water. A chemical reaction identifies a relationship between reactants and products. Products will be formed during a reaction and identified on the right side of the equation. Catalysts can be used to speed up a reaction or cause a reaction, however they are never destroyed.

Thermodynamics

Endothermic reactions are reactions that absorb energy. Exothermic reactions are reactions that give off energy/heat.

1st Law of Thermodynamics-energy is conserved with every process.
2nd Law of Thermodynamics-the total entropy of a chemical system and that of its area always increases if the chemical or physical change is spontaneous.
Entropy is defined as the quantity of disorder in a chemical environment.

> ➤ **Review Video: <u>Laws of Thermodynamics</u>**
> *Visit **mometrix.com/academy** and enter **Code: 253607***

Temperature Conversions:

Kelvin (K) = Celsius degree +273.15

Fahrenheit (F) = (9/5 (Celsius)) +32

Kinetic Theory of Energy- all atoms are in constant motion

Gases obey the following laws:

Charles law (Gay Lussac's law)-volume of a gas varies indirectly with temperature with pressure constant.
V/T = constant

Boyle's law-volume of a gas varies inversely with pressure if temperature is constant.
The two common units of Pressure (P) are atmosphere and Mercury millimeters.
1 atm = 760 mm Hg
PV = constant

Avogadro's law –equal volumes of all gases contain the same number of molecules.
Avogadro's number- 6.02×10^{23}.

Ideal Gas Equation
PV = nRT

Newton's Laws of Motion

1st Law- (Law of Inertia) - A moving object will resist any change in velocity. A resting object with resist any change to begin moving.

> ➤ **Review Video: Newton's 1st Law of Motion**
> *Visit* ***mometrix.com/academy*** *and enter* ***Code: 590367***

2nd Law- (Force = Mass x Acceleration, F=ma) – An object's acceleration is determined by the sum of the forces on the object divided by the object's mass.

> ➤ **Review Video: Newton's 2nd Law of Motion**
> *Visit* ***mometrix.com/academy*** *and enter* ***Code: 737975***

3rd Law- An equal and opposite reaction force is generated when a force is applied to an object. The object with greater mass will generally absorb the force without any discernible acceleration.

> ➤ **Review Video: Newton's 3rd Law of Motion**
> *Visit* ***mometrix.com/academy*** *and enter* ***Code: 838401***

Velocity is the rate of change of position. Acceleration is the rate of change of velocity.

Waves

Wavelength- the distance between the highest points of a wave
Amplitude- half of the height of a wave, from the top of a crest to the bottom of a trough
Key Formulas

Momentum = Mass x Velocity

Acceleration = $\dfrac{\text{Change in Velocity}}{\text{Total Time}}$

Speed = $\dfrac{\text{Distance}}{\text{Time}}$

Work=Force x Distance

Power= $\dfrac{\text{F x D}}{\text{T}}$

Power= Voltage x Current
Watts=Voltage x Amperes

Ohm's law, V = I*R

I = current
V = potential difference
R = resistance

Resistance in a Parallel circuit: $1/Rt = 1/R1 + 1/R2 + 1/R3 +...$
Resistance in a Series circuit: $Rt = R1 + R2 + R3$
Rt = R (t)otal

Backtrack for Units
When faced with a problem that you don't know the formula for, simply solve for the units in the answer choices. The units in the answer choices are your key to understanding what mathematical relationship exists between the numbers given in the question.
Example: A 600 Hz sound wave has a velocity of 160 m/s. What is the wavelength of this sound wave?

Even if you do not know the formula for wavelengths, you can backtrack to get the answer by using the units in the answer choices. The answer choices are:
    A. 0.17 m
    B. 0.27 m
    C. 0.35 m
    D. 0.48 m
You know that Hz is equal to 1/s. To get an answer in m, when working with a m/s and a 1/s from the problem, you must divide the m/s by 1/s, which will leave an answer in meters or m. Therefore (160 m/s) / (600 1/s) = .27 m, making choice B correct.

Don't Fall for the Obvious
When in doubt of the answer, it is easy to go with what you are familiar with. If you recognize only one term in four answer choices, you may be inclined to guess at that term. Be careful though, and don't go with familiar answers simply because they are familiar.
Example: Changing the temperature of the solution to 373K would most likely result in:
    A. boiling the solution
    B. freezing the solution
    C. dissolving the compound
    D. saturating the solution
You know that 373K is the boiling point of pure water. Therefore choice A is familiar, because you have a mental link between the temperature 373K and the

word "boiling". If you are unsure of the correct answer, you may decide upon choice A simply because of its familiarity. Don't be deceived though. Think through the other answer choices before making your final selection. Just because you have a mental link between two terms, doesn't make an answer choice correct.

Milk the Question
Some of the questions may throw you completely off. They might deal with a subject you have not been exposed to, or one that you haven't reviewed in years. While your lack of knowledge about the subject will be a hindrance, the question itself can give you many clues that will help you find the correct answer. Read the question carefully, and look for clues. Watch particularly for adjectives and nouns describing difficult terms or words that you don't recognize. Regardless of if you understand a word or not, replacing it with the synonyms used for it in the question may help you to understand what the questions are asking.
Example: A bacteriophage is a virus that infects bacteria....

While you may not know much information concerning the characteristics of a bacteriophage, the fifth word into the sentence told you that a bacteriophage is a virus. Whenever a question asks about a bacteriophage, you can mentally replace the word "bacteriophage" with the word "virus". Your more general knowledge of viruses will enable you to answer the question intelligibly.

Look carefully for these descriptive synonyms (nouns) and adjectives and use them to help you understand the difficult terms. Rather than wracking your mind about specific detail information concerning a difficult term in the question, use the more general description or synonym provided to make it easier for you.

Work Fast
Since you have 60 questions to answer in only 60 minutes, that means that you have 1 minute to spend per question. This section faces a greater time crunch that any other test you will take on the RN Pre-entrance exam, for though the Verbal Test also has a 1 minute per question time restriction, the questions in the Science Test may sometimes have calculations associated with them that could require more time. While the Mathematics Test allows 1.5 minutes for these calculation questions, there is no such luxury for the Science Test. Therefore, if you are stuck on one word, don't waste too much time. Eliminate the answers you could bet a quick $5 on and then pick the first one that remains. You can make a note in your book and if you have time you can always come back, but don't waste your time. You have to work fast!

Random Tips

- On fact questions that require choosing between numbers, don't guess the smallest or largest choice unless you're sure of the answer (remember- "sure" means you would bet $5 on it).
- For questions that you're not clear on the answer, use the process of elimination. Weed out the answer choices that you know are wrong before choosing an answer.
- Don't fall for "bizarre" choices, mentioning things that are not relevant to the passage. Also avoid answers that sound "smart." Again, if you're willing to bet $5, ignore the tips and go with your bet.

Practice Test

Verbal Review

1. The data in the graph exhibited an *aberration*.
   Aberration means:

   A: deviation from course
   B: linear appearance
   C: inverted appearance
   D: circular theme

2. The prince *abjured* the ambassador.
   Abjured means:

   A: congratulated
   B: renounced
   C: relieved
   D: fired

3. The chemist attempted to practice *alchemy*.
   Alchemy means:

   A: turning metal into gold
   B: separating ions
   C: fusion
   D: isolating chemical components

4. The man at the bar was *belligerent*.
   Belligerent means:

   A: friendly
   B: courteous
   C: angry
   D: talkative

5. The ships formed a *blockade* near the mouth of the Mississippi River.
   Blockade means:

   A: prevent passage
   B: fishing convoy
   C: whaling expedition
   D: zigzag formation

6. The men erected a *bulwark* near the opening.
   Bulwark means:

A: trap
B: obstacle
C: barn
D: runway

7. The group embarked on a *clandestine* operation.
   Clandestine means:

A: environmental expedition
B: shipping adventure
C: scary
D: secretive

8. The agent of the government was *choleric*.
   Choleric means:

A: easily provoked
B: undercover
C: cooperative
D: late

9. Some members of the organization broke away and created a grass roots *caucus*.
   Caucus means:

A: group with political aims
B: environmental group
C: management organization
D: religious movement

10. The circumstancess were open to *conjecture*.
    Conjecture means:

A: discussion
B: guessing
C: argument
D: public

11. The news anchor attempted to *disseminate* the story.
    Disseminate means:

A: to convey
B: to deny
C: to rebuke
D: to review

12. The stockpiles for the occupation began to *dwindle*.
    Dwindle means:

A: to increase
B: to decrease
C: to rot
D: to be self-limiting

13. The chemicals began to *effervesce*.
    Effervesce means:

A: to combine
B: to catalyze
C: to break down
D: to bubble up

14. The witness began to *evince* critical details.
    Evince means:

A: to hide
B: to cover secretly
C: exaggerate
D: to make manifest

15. The front line troops began to *extricate* from the enemy.
    Extricate means:

A: confront
B: surrender
C: disentangle
D: deploy

16. The congressman from Ohio started a *filibuster*.
    Filibuster means:

A: bill
B: congressional investigation
C: an attempt to disrupt legislation
D: program related to welfare

17. The soldier showed *fortitude* during the engagement with the enemy.
    Fortitude means:

A: patient courage
B: willingness for action
C: endurance
D: professionalism

18. The southern lady was *genteel* when hosting northern businessmen.
    Genteel means:

A: rude
B: refined
C: reserved
D: resentful

19. The lawyer launched into a *harangue* when speaking to the witness.
    Harangue means:

A: discussion
B: monologue
C: dialogue
D: tirade

20. Some believe our destinies are *immutable*.
    Immutable means:

A: professional
B: conversational
C: unchangeable
D: unerring

21. The baby was diagnosed with *jaundice*.
    Jaundice means:

A: yellowing condition
B: condition of glucose intolerance
C: condition of nutritional deficiency
D: condition of dermatitis

22. The criminal was known for his *knavery*.
    Knavery means:

A: quickness
B: light-footedness
C: burglary ability
D: deceitfulness

23. The patient exhibited signs of *languor*.
    Languor means:

A: confusion
B: anxiety
C: depression
D: deceitfulness

24. The Romans were able to *macadamize* a large portion of the Italian peninsula.
    Macadamize means:

A: to pave
B: to supply
C: to connect
D: to protect

25. The patient's lower extremity began to show signs of *necrosis*.
    Necrosis means:

A: maceration
B: tissue death
C: induration
D: redness

26. The traffic official began to *obviate* the construction.
    Obviate means:

A: clear away
B: identify
C: reproduce
D: delegate

27. The general *presaged* the battle plan to his subordinate officers.
    Presaged means:

A: delegated
B: clarified
C: foretold
D: introduced

28. The orange grove was under *quarantine*, because of a local virus.
    Quarantine means:

A: pressure
B: demolition
C: reconstruction
D: isolation

29. The defendant was asked to *remunerate* the damage he caused during the
    robbery.
    Remunerate means:

A: reconstruct
B: renounce
C: pay for
D: repeat

30. The welding machine *scintillated* into the dark shop.
    Scintillated means:

A: emitted gases
B: emitted light
C: emitted fumes
D: emitted noise

31. The mission was *surreptitious* in nature.
    Surreptitious means:

A: transforming
B: dangerous
C: invasive
D: secret

32. The desert conditions were *torrid* for the Israeli division operating in the Sinai.
    Torrid means:

A: excessively hot
B: aggravating
C: lukewarm
D: inhospitable

33. The adventurer left with a feeling of *trepidation*.
    Trepidation means:

A: uncertainty
B: extreme depression
C: ambivalence
D: fearfulness

34. The fish exhibited an *unctuous* appearance at the fish market.
    Unctuous means:

A: fresh
B: dirty
C: oily
D: lucid

35. The venal politician preyed upon his constituents during his time in office.
    Venal means:

A: barbaric
B: current
C: ambivalent
D: corrupt

Mathematics Review
(no calculator)

36.   897.54 – 48.39 =

A: 849.15
B: 813.15
C: 859.15
D: 814.15

37.   1053.33 – 545.69 =

A: 519.64
B: 517.54
C: 508.64
D: 507.64

38.   893.42 + 82.77 =

A: 976.09
B: 976.29
C: 986.19
D: 976.19

39.   94.31 + 973.37 =

A: 1067.68
B: 1167.68
C: 1067.78
D: 1167.78

40.   A senior paid $3.47, $9.50 and $2.50 for lunch during a basketball
       tournament. What was the average amount he paid over three days?

A: $5.18
B: $5.25
C: $5.16
D: $5.37

41.   89.35 x 32.75 =

A: 2826.23
B: 2925.31
C: 2926.21
D: 2837.41

42.   Using the following equation, solve for (x). 3x – 4y = 25 and (y)=2

A: x =10
B: x = 11
C: x = 12
D: x = 13

43.   Using the following equation, solve for (y). 5y – 3x = 24 and (x) = 7

A: y = 8
B: y = 9
C: y = 10
D: y = 11

44.   An armoire was purchased for $340.32 at an auction, subject to a 5% tax rate. What was the additional tax charged on the armoire?

A: $15.82
B: $16.02
C: $16.39
D: $17.02

45.   894 + ((3)(12)) =

A: 730
B: 932
C: 930
D: 945

46.   Round to the nearest 2 decimal places, 892/15 =

A: 60.47
B: 59.47
C: 62.57
D: 59.57

47.   Round to the nearest 2 decimal places, 999.52/13 =

A: 76.89
B: 76.97
C: 86.87
D: 86.97

48.   Round to the nearest 2 decimal places, 9.42/3.47 =

A: 2.63
B: 2.71
C: 2.81
D: 2.94

49.   Jonathan Edwards ate 8.32 lbs. of food over 3 days. What was his average
        intake?

A: 2.66 lbs.
B: 2.77 lbs.
C: 2.87 lbs.
D: 2.97 lbs.

50.   Which of the following decimals equals 9.47%?

A: .000947
B: .00947
C: .0947
D: .9470

51.   .10 equals which of the following fractions?

A: 1/100
B: 1/10
C: 1/50
D: 1/5

52.   What is the area of a rectangle with sides 34 meters and 12 meters?

A: 408
B: 2.83
C: 22
D: 40.8

53.   The standard ratio of (number of treatments) and (total mL dose) is 3.5 to 2
        mL. If only 2 treatments are given, how many total mL doses are given?

A: 1.58 mL
B: 2.34 mL
C: 1.14 mL
D: 2.58 mL

54. If one side of a triangle equals 4 inches and the second side equals 5 inches, what does the third side equal?

A: 9 inches
B: 1 inches
C: 6.4 inches
D: 4.6 inches

55. If $x=75 + 0$, and $y= (75)(0)$, then

A: x>y
B: x=y
C: x<y
D: x+y = 0

56. If $x=3$, the $x^2+x=$

A: 9
B: 15
C: 12
D: 10

57. If $a=4$ and $b=5$, then $a (a^2+b)=$

A: 52
B: 84
C: 62
D: 64

58. If $x= ¼, y=1/2$, and $z= 2/3$, then $x +y- z =$

A: 1/8
B: 2/9
C: 1/12
D: 2/5

59. If $x= ½, y=1/3, z=3/8$, then $x(y-z)=$

A: 1/48
B: -1/48
C: 1/64
D: -1/64

60:    2/3 cup of oil is needed for a cake recipe, and you have 1/4 cup. How much more oil do you need?

A: 1/2
B: 2/7
C: 3/8
D: 5/12

61:    8 ¾ + 6 ½ =

A: 32
B: 15 ¼
C: 14 ½
D: 17 ¾

62.   A senior citizen was billed $ 3.85 for a long-distance phone call. The first 10 minutes cost $3.50, and 35 cents was charged for each additional minute. How long was the telephone call?

A: 17 minutes
B: 20 minutes
C: 15 minutes
D: 11 minutes

63.   A ½ cup of skim milk is 45 calories. Approximately how many calories would ¾ cup of skim milk provide?

A: 67 ½
B: 68
C: 76 ½
D: 60

64. $10b = 5a - 15$. If $a = 3$, then $b =$

A: 7
B: 5
C: 1
D: 0

65.   (5 x 4) ÷ (2 x 2) =

A: 6
B: 7.2
C: 5
D: 4

66.   Which of these numbers is a prime number?

A: 12
B: 4
C: 15
D: 11

67.   12 members of a weight loss club are female; there are 23 members altogether. Approximately what percentage of members are males?

A: 59%
B: 48%
C: 36%
D: 44%

68.   A person travels an average of 57 miles daily, and this morning he traveled 14 miles. What percentage of his daily average of mile traveled did he travel this morning?

A: 25%
B: 22%
C: 27%
D: 32%

69.   75 is 60% of what number?

A: 130
B: 125
C: 45
D: 145

70.   A student invests $3000 of his student loan and receives 400 dollars in interest over a 4-year period. What is his average yearly interest rate?

A: 3.3%
B: 2.1%
C: 5%
D: 4.2%

Science Review

71.   The heart is divided into __ chambers.

A: 2
B: 3
C: 4
D: 5

72.   Blood leaves the right ventricle and goes to the ____.

A: lungs
B: kidneys
C: right atrium
D: arterial circulation to the body

73.   Which of the following does not help determine heart rate?

A: body temperature
B: physical activity
C: concentration of ions
D: anaerobic cellular metabolism

74.   Which of the following is not considered a layer of the heart?

A: epicardium
B: endocarcium
C: myocardium
D: vasocardium

75.   The hormone _____ can promote increased blood volume, and increased blood pressure.

A: estrogen
B: testosterone
C: aldosterone
D: dopamine

76.   Which of the following terms matches the definition: an abnormally slow heartbeat.

A: tachycardia
B: bradycardia
C: fibrillation
D: myocardial infarct

- 84 -

77. Blood is made of approximately ___% hematocrit and ____% plasma.

A: 45, 55
B: 55, 45
C: 75, 25
D: 25, 75

78. The right lung has ___ lobes and the left lung has ___ lobes.

A: 2, 3
B: 3, 2
C: 4, 2
D: 2, 4

79. Aerobic respiration in cells occurs in the _____.

A: cytoplasm
B: nucleus
C: mitochondria
D: cell membrane

80. Which of the following terms matches the definition: collapse of a lung.

A: anoxia
B: atelectasis
C: dyspnea
D: hypercapnia

81. The central nervous system is composed of the _____ and the _____.

A: brain, spinal cord
B: brain, peripheral nerves
C: spinal cord, peripheral nerves
D: spinal cord, musculature system

82. The brain is made of _____ lobes.

A: 2
B: 3
C: 4
D: 5

83. _____ is a state of equilibrium within tissues.

A: peristalsis
B: somatitis
C: homeostasis
D: synergy

84. _____ is a state of inflammation of the mouth.

A: diverticulitis
B: hepatitis
C: enteritis
D: somatitis

85. _____ is the most important male hormone

A: estrogen
B: aldosterone
C: progesterone
D: testosterone

86. Which of the following functions are not related to the kidneys?

A: filtration
B: bile production
C: secretion
D: re-absorption

87. Which of the following terms matches the definition: uncontrolled urination.

A: enuresis
B: dieuretic
C: pyuria
D: ureteritis

88. Auditory impulses are interpreted in the _____ lobes.

A: frontal
B: parietal
C: temporal
D: occipital

89.   The outer layer of the eye is the ____.

A: cornea
B: sclera
C: retina
D: rods

90.   The inner layer of the eye is the ____.

A: cornea
B: sclera
C: retina
D: rods

91.   Which of the following elements are not halogens?

A: Chlorine
B: Bromide
C: Iodine
D: Cesium

92.   The horizontal rows of the periodic table are called ____.

A: periods
B: columns
C: rows
D: families

93   A/an ____ is the simplest unit of an element.

A: atom
B: molecule
C: electron
D: neutron

94.   Compounds with various structures, but the same shape are called ____.

A: polar compounds
B: isomers
C: variables
D: transient compounds

95.   Converting gas into a liquid is known as _____.

A: evaporation
B: transitioning
C: condensation
D: sublimation

96.   Which of the following terms matches the definition: the volume of a gas varies indirectly with temperature with pressure constant.

A: Boyle's law
B: Charles law
C: Johnson's law
D: Avogadro's law

97.   Which of the following terms matches the definition: energy is conserved with every process.

A: 1st Law of Thermodynamics
B: 2nd Law of Thermodynamics
C: 3rd Law of Thermodynamics
D: 4th Law of Thermodynamics

98.   An acid is a substance that increases the _____ count in water.

A: chloride ion
B: hydroxide ion
C: hydrogen ion
D: oxygen

99.   Which of the following is not true of a reaction catalyst's potential?

A: it can speed up a reaction
B: it can cause a reaction
C: it is never destroyed
D: it is always found on the right side of an equation

100.   Using the 2nd Law of Newton identify the formula that is applicable.

A: F=ma
B: Speed = $\frac{Distance}{Time}$
C: Power = $\frac{F \times D}{T}$
D: Watts = Voltage x Amperes

- 88 -

Answer Key

Number	Answer	Number	Answer	Number	Answer	Number	Answer
1	A	26	A	51	B	76	B
2	B	27	C	52	A	77	A
3	A	28	D	53	C	78	B
4	C	29	C	54	C	79	C
5	A	30	B	55	A	80	B
6	B	31	D	56	C	81	A
7	D	32	A	57	B	82	C
8	A	33	D	58	C	83	C
9	A	34	C	59	B	84	D
10	B	35	D	60	D	85	D
11	A	36	A	61	B	86	B
12	B	37	D	62	D	87	A
13	D	38	D	63	A	88	C
14	D	39	A	64	D	89	B
15	C	40	C	65	C	90	C
16	C	41	C	66	D	91	D
17	A	42	B	67	B	92	A
18	B	43	B	68	A	93	A
19	D	44	D	69	B	94	B
20	C	45	C	70	A	95	C
21	A	46	B	71	C	96	B
22	D	47	A	72	A	97	A
23	C	48	B	73	D	98	C
24	A	49	B	74	D	99	D
25	B	50	C	75	C	100	A

Answer Explanations
Verbal Review

1. A: Aberration means a deviation from what is normal or typical. Its Latin roots are ab-, meaning away from, and errare, meaning to err or stray. Combined, these make up the Latin verb aberrare, to go astray (from). There are no other meanings.

2. B: To abjure means "to renounce." The original Latin roots are ab-, meaning away from, and jurare, meaning to swear, which is also the root of the English word jury. Hence "swearing away from" is renouncing, rejecting, or repudiating someone or something, abstaining from or avoiding something, or taking something back.

3. A: Alchemy refers to the hypothetical process of turning base metals into gold. While this process does not exist in reality, it was a famously popular pursuit during the Middle Ages. Today this word is also used figuratively to mean turning something common into something precious, or any mysterious transformation. The Medieval Latin alchymia derived from the Arabic al-kimiya, originating from the Late Greek word chemeia.

4. C: Belligerent means angry or hostile. Its original sense had to do with waging war. Belligerare in Latin means "to wage war," from bellum, which means war (as in the English word "antebellum," meaning prewar), and gerare, which means to wage. "Hostilities" in English can refer to warfare and to anger. An English synonym of belligerent from the same root is "bellicose." Both mean warlike, aggressive, combative, etc.

5. A: Blockade refers to preventing passage or blocking it. Its similarity to the word "block" makes it easier to define. One difference between "block" and "blockade" is that "blockade" was originally, and is still often, used to refer specifically to military maneuvers intended to block physically the transportation, trade, and communications of enemy nations. It also refers to obstruction of physiological processes and, generally, to any obstruction. It can be used as a transitive verb or a noun.

6. B: The choice closest to the meaning of bulwark is obstacle. A bulwark is a protective, defensive, or supportive structure that is like a wall. Synonyms include rampart, breakwater, and seawall. The (usually) plural term "bulwarks" can also refer to a ship's sides above the upper deck. It is also used abstractly, as in "Democratic ideals provide a bulwark against despotism."

7. D: The adjective clandestine means secretive or in secret. The Latin source word clandestinus derived from clam, meaning secretly. Secret, and synonyms like covert, furtive, undercover, stealthy, surreptitious, etc., represent the only meaning of this word.

8. A: Choleric means easily provoked. Synonyms include hot-tempered, irate, irritable, angry, etc. In ancient Greek civilization, Hippocrates and other physicians subscribed to the theory that the body contained four essential substances they called humors: blood, phlegm (mucus), yellow bile, and black bile, which should be balanced. The physician Galen named four temperaments resulting from unbalanced dominance of one humor: sanguine with blood, phlegmatic with mucus, melancholic with yellow bile, and choleric with black bile. This is the origin of the word and its meaning.

9. A: A caucus is a group with political aims. For example, the National Women's Political Caucus, the National Black Caucus, the National Caucus of Environmental Legislators, the Tea Party Caucus, etc. The origin of this word is unknown. It can mean a closed group meeting of members of a political party or faction to make policy decisions or choose candidates, or a group promoting a cause. There are no other meanings.

10. B: Conjecture means guessing or speculation. Synonyms include supposition, inference, and surmise. The Latin conjectura is the past participle of the verb conicere, meaning literally to throw together. The English word is a noun. It has no alternate meanings.

11. A: The closest choice is "to convey." Disseminate means to spread or distribute, or to disperse throughout, as is done when sowing seeds. Indeed, the Latin root of this word is semen, which means "seed" in English and is the English biological term for male spermatic fluid, i.e., human or animal "seed."

12. B: To dwindle means "to decrease," usually steadily. It can be a transitive or intransitive verb, e.g., to make less or to become less. It is thought to originate from the Old English verb dwinan, to waste away, probably derived from the Old Norse words dvina, to pine away, and/or deyja, to die. This word has no alternate definitions.

13. D: To bubble up is a synonym for "to effervesce." The related adjective is effervescent, meaning bubbly—literally as in bubbly liquids, or figuratively, as in bubbly personalities. The origin is the Latin verb fervere, meaning "to boil." The formatives ex- meaning out, and fervescere, meaning to begin to boil, combined to produce effervescere, meaning to effervesce or boil out, as when steam escapes.

14. D: Evince means "to make manifest or demonstrate." Other synonyms include: to show, display, or reveal. The Latin verb vincere means to conquer (e.g., Julius Caesar's "Veni, vidi, vici" meaning "I came, I saw, I conquered"). Derived from this is evincere, to vanquish or win a point.

15. C: Disentangle is the best choice as a synonym for extricate. It means to remove from entanglement, or to differentiate from something related. Its roots are the

- 91 -

Latin ex-, meaning out, and tricae, meaning trifles or perplexities. These combine to form the verb extricare, whose past participle is extricatus.

16. C: A filibuster is an attempt to disrupt legislation. In United States government, it commonly takes the form of engaging in a lengthy speech on the floor of the Senate, House of Representatives, state legislature, and so on, to delay or prevent voting to pass a law or similar actions. This word's origin, the Spanish filibustero, meaning freebooter, is also the source of its other meaning: an irregular military adventurer, specifically an American inciting rebellion in 1850s Latin America. These are the only two definitions.

17. A: Fortitude refers to strength of mind or of character that enables someone to have courage in the face of adversity. Its root is the same as the words "fort" and "fortify." Fort means strong in French. All these come from the Latin fortis, also meaning strong. (In Shakespeare's play Hamlet, the name of the supporting character Fortinbras transliterates to "strong in arm" in English.) If you chose "endurance" as the answer, this is understandable, as one can "endure" hardship; however, endurance refers more to lasting a long time, wearing well, etc., related to durable and duration, from Latin durare, to harden or last, from durus, or hard, rather than referring to strength. The original meaning of fortitude was simply strength, now considered obsolete, superseded by the current definition of non-physical strength.

18. B: Genteel means refined and comes from the French gentil, meaning gentle, as in gentilhomme, for gentleman. It can mean aristocratic, polite, elegant, or related to the gentry or upper class. Other meanings are connected with appearing or trying to appear socially superior or respectable; being falsely delicate, prudish, or affected; or being conventionally and/or ineffectually pretty, as in artistic style.

19. D: A tirade is the nearest synonym to a harangue. A harangue can simply mean a speech addressing a public assembly. It can also mean a lecture. A third meaning, most commonly used in contemporary English, is a spoken or written rant. While a monologue is also delivered by one person, it does not include the ranting connotations of harangue and tirade. Diatribe and philippic are other synonyms.

20. C: Immutable means unchangeable. The Latin verb mutare means to change. Its past participle is mutates, the root of the English verb "mutate" and noun "mutation," as used in biology when genes or viruses mutate, or change in form or characteristics.

21. A: Jaundice is a yellowing condition. The French adjective jaune means yellow. The Latin root for the French and English words is galbinus, or greenish-yellow. When people or animals develop jaundice, their skin and the whites of their eyes turn yellowish. Jaundice is usually due to liver damage or dysfunction; the yellow color comes from a buildup of bile. This word is also used figuratively to mean a

feeling of distaste, hostility, or being fed up, as in "a jaundiced attitude" or "a jaundiced view" of something or someone.

22. D: Deceitfulness is closest to knavery in meaning. In the Middle Ages, a roguish, rascally, mischievous, or tricky, deceitful fellow was called a knave. The Jack in a deck of playing cards was also formerly called the Knave. This Middle English word derived from the Old English cnafa.

23. C: The closest choice to languor is depression. Languor means listlessness, apathy, inertia, slowness, sluggishness, or weakness/weariness of the body or mind. The related adjective is "languid." The root is Latin.

24. A: Macadamize means "to pave." The related word "macadam" refers to paving material. It originates from the name of John L. McAdam, a nineteenth-century Scottish engineer who turned road construction into a science and invented the process of macadamization. Over time, macadamize and macadam have evolved to refer to a variety of processes and materials for building roads.

25. B: Necrosis refers to tissue death. It shares roots with words like necropsy, necrophilia, and so on. The original root is the Greek nekros, meaning dead body. The "necro-" root is used in medical terminology and refers to death.

26. A: Preclude is the only synonym for obviate among these choices. To obviate means to prevent, avert, or forestall; or to render unnecessary. Both meanings incorporate the element of anticipating something in advance. The root is the Latin verb obviare, which meant to meet or withstand; the past participle is obviatus.

27. C: Presaged means foretold. You may recognize the Latin prefix pre-, meaning before. The Latin root word sagus means prophetic, which is also the root of the English word "seek." Presage can be a verb or a noun.

28. D: Quarantine means isolation. Quadraginta is the original Latin root. Quarantine developed from the Latinate languages French, whose quarante means forty, and Italian, with its cognate quaranta. It was a custom in the seventeenth century to isolate ships for 40 days to prevent diseases and pests from spreading. In fact, another definition of quarantine is a 40-day period.

29. C: To remunerate means to pay for something, as in remunerating someone's services or paying someone. Synonyms include to pay, to compensate, or to recompense. In Latin, munus means gift. The verb for this noun is munerare, to give. Combined with re- for back, remunerare is to give back, and its past participle is remuneratus, the root of remunerate.

30. B: To scintillate is to emit light—literally, to sparkle. The Latin noun scintilla means spark. This word is also in the English vocabulary. The Latin verb "to sparkle"

is scintillare; its past participle is scintillatus, the English word's root. The adjective "scintillating" is commonly used figuratively to describe a sparkling personality, conversation, or witticism.

31. D: Surreptitious means secret. Other common synonyms are stealthy, covert, and clandestine. The root is Latin surrepticius, the past participle of surripere, to snatch secretly, a verb combined from sub- (under) and rapere (to seize).

32. A: Torrid means excessively hot, scorching; or parched with heat, especially from the sun. The root is Latin torridus, from the verb torrere, to roast. In physical geography, the Torrid Zone is the name for the central latitude zone of the earth, between the Tropic of Cancer and the Tropic of Capricorn, where temperatures are hottest.

33. D: Trepidation means fearfulness. Synonyms include apprehension, anxiety, dread, alarm, fear, terror, and horror. It comes from the Latin verb trepidare, to tremble; the adjective trepidus means agitated.

34. C: Unctuous means oily, or fatty. It also means greasy and smooth in texture, or plastic, that is, malleable. A third meaning is figuratively "oily," as in someone whose manner is falsely earnest, ingratiating, and/or smug. This figurative meaning is often used by literary authors. The Latin root is unguere, to anoint. The noun "unction", used for the figurative meaning and in religion, has the same root.

35. D: Venal means corrupt, or corruptible, that is, capable of being bought. Its root is the Latin venalis, from venum, meaning sale. Other synonyms are bribable, purchasable, mercenary, or dirty.

Mathematics Review

36. A: The correct remainder is 849.15. When subtracting numbers with a decimal point, you borrow the same way as you do when there is no decimal. Thus the first digits to the left of the decimal are 7 – 8; you borrow 1 from the 9 to the left of the 7, making the 7 into 17. 17 – 8 = 9. The borrowed-from 9 becomes an 8; 8 – 4 = 4.

37. D: The correct remainder is 507.64. When subtracting larger digits from smaller ones, you must borrow from the next digit to the left, adding a 1 to the smaller digit. In the decimal system, the borrowed 1 adds a unit of 10 to the digit to make it >10— big enough to subtract any digit from 1 to 9 in the subtrahend from it. Hence the rightmost 3 in the minuend borrows 1 from the 3 to its left, making it 13. 13 – 9 = 4. The borrowed-from 3 becomes 2. You borrow 1 from the 3 to the left; 12 – 6 = 6; etc. Borrowing continues across the decimal point in numbers with decimals.

38. D: The correct sum is 976.19. When adding numbers with decimal points, you add them the same way as numbers with no decimal. Thus, adding the 7 + 4 to the right of the decimal point, the sum is 11; you write 1 and then carry the other 1 to

- 94 -

the left of the decimal point. So 3 + 2 + carried 1 = 6. Two places left of the decimal, 8 + 9 = 17; write 7 and carry the 1; so 8 + carried 1 = 9.

39. A: The correct sum is 1076.68. When adding numbers with a decimal point in any place in which the sum is >10, you write down the right-hand digit and carry the left-hand digit over to the next place to the left. Thus, when adding the 7 two places to the left of the decimal in 973.37 with the 9 in 94.31, 7 + 9 = 16, so you write down a 6 and carry the 1 to the next place, where 9 + 1 = 10.

40. C: This word problem requires an average. You add $3.47 + $9.50 + $2.50. This equals $15.47. Since there were three amounts, you then divide $15.47 by 3, and the result is $5.1567. When working with amounts of money, you round off anything beyond two digits to the right of the decimal to get a usable number of cents. If the third digit to the right is 1 through 4, you ignore it and leave the second digit as is. If the third digit is 5 or more, you round the second digit up, as in this case; so $5.1567 becomes $5.16.

41. C: The correct product is 2926.21. When multiplying numbers with multiple digits, you first multiply every digit in the multiplicand respectively by the rightmost digit in the multiplier; then by the multiplier's second digit to the left, then by the third, and so on. You write each product below and one place to the left of the previous product, and add all products together. First, multiply 89.35 by the 5 in 32.75, getting 446.75. Then multiply 89.35 by the 7 in 32.75, getting 625.45, which you write below and one place to the left of 446.75. 89.35 x 2 = 178.70, written below and one place to the left of 625.45. 89.35 x 3 = 286.05, written below and one place to the left of 178.70. Temporarily removing the decimal points may make it easier to add the staggered columns, replacing the point in the final summed product:

```
        8935
    x   3275
       44675

       62545
       17870
       28605
     29262125
```

After multiplying two numbers with two decimal places each, 2 x 2 = 4, so place the decimal point 4 places from the end, = 2926.2125. Discard the final 25 = 2926.21.

42. B: In this equation, the unknown quantity is (x). (y) = 2. In the equation, substitute 2 for y: 3x − 4*2 = 25. 4y, or 4*2 = 8. So 3x − 8 = 25. If 25 is the remainder of 3x − 8, add 8 back to 25: 25 + 8 = 33. This means that 3x = 33. 33 ÷ 3 = 11. Therefore, x = 11.

43. B: In this equation, (x) = 7 and (y) is unknown. 3x = 3*7 = 21. Therefore, 5y – 21 = 24. It follows that if 5y – 21 = 24, then 24 + 21 = 5y. 24 + 21 = 45, so 45 = 5y. 45 / 5 = 9, so (y) = 9.

44. D: To determine the tax, you must calculate 5% of $340.32. 5% = .05. So you multiply $340.32 by .05, getting $17.0160. When multiplying two numbers, each with two decimal places, you also multiply the decimal places, so the product has four places right of the point. Since you want cents here, you eliminate the final (rightmost) zero; the digit 6 rounds up the 1 left of it to a 2, and is then discarded, yielding a final product of $17.02.

45. C: First, multiply the two multiples, (3)(12). 3*12 = 36. Then add 894 + 36. The sum is 930. Whenever two or more figures are in parentheses as they are here, this means the operation (in this case, multiplication) with these figures is performed first. The operation outside of the parentheses (in this case, addition) is performed afterward on the result of the first operation.

46. B: With 892 ÷ 15, you get 59.4666, and so on (you will get an endless recurrence of 6 in the last place if you continue to divide). The convention with digits > 5 is to round up to the next higher number. Since this problem specifies to the nearest two decimal places, you round .46 up to .47.

47. A: 999.52 ÷ 13 yields 76.886 (with many more digits continuing to the right before getting to an even quotient with nothing left over to be divided further). The convention is to round up digits > 5. So rounding to the nearest two decimal places, 76.88 is rounded up to 76.89 because the third digit was a 6.

48. B: 9.42 ÷ 3.47 gives a quotient of 2.714697 followed by many more digits before reaching an even division. Since the third decimal place has a 4, you do not round the second decimal place up because only half of 10 or more, i.e., > 5, will round up the next decimal place. Since 4 < 5, the 1 is left as is, yielding 2.71.

49. B: To get the average, divide the 8.32 pounds of food by the 3 days. 8.32/3 = 2.773333..... Since you will keep getting a 3 by continuing to divide, and 3 < 5, you do not round up the previous decimal places. Rounding off to two decimal places, the average = 2.77 pounds.

50. C: The correct version is .0947. An even 9% = .09 because percentages are per 100; the first decimal place equals tenths, the second equals hundreds, and so on. When we use the % sign, we eliminate the decimal point and any leading zeros as redundant. We write either .09 or 9%. So, since 9% already equals 9/100 or .09, in the figure 9.47, the .47 represents 47 hundredths of a percent. 9% does not equal the whole number 9; it equals 9/100. Decimal points are not repeated within one number. Instead, each successive decimal place equals another tenth (tens,

- 96 -

hundreds, thousands, ten-thousands, hundred-thousands, millions, et cetera) Therefore, 9-and-47-hundredths percent = .0947.

51. B: .10 equals 1/10. In the decimal system, whole numbers are left of the decimal point. One decimal place (to the right of the point) = tenths; two places = hundredths; three places = thousandths, and so on. 1/100 would be .010; 1/50 would be .02; and 1/5 would be .20.

52. A: To obtain the area of a rectangle, multiply the two lengths of the sides: 34 meters * 12 meters = 408 meters.

53. C: The standard ratio given is 3.5 treatments : 2 milliliters. To find out how many milliliters are in one dose, $2 \div 3.5 = 0.57$ of a milliliter. If only two doses are given, multiply 0.57 ml * 2 = 1.14 total milliliters given.

54. C: An obtuse triangle has one angle >90°. An acute triangle has all angles <90°. With a 4" side and a 5" side, the third side must be either >5" or <4" for it to be an obtuse triangle. 1" is too short: the sides could not meet unless they were parallel, that is, a 180° angle. 9" is too long to connect with 4" and 5" sides; at the widest possible angle, the 4" side would still be too short to meet the others. 4.6" is in between 4" and 5", so this makes an acute angle; therefore, the triangle would be acute, not obtuse. 6.4" is longer than the 5" side (the longer of the two sides given), so the angle is >90° and is therefore obtuse.

55. A: This problem illustrates the property of zero and the identity property. Any number + 0 = the same number, so 75 + 0 = 75. Any number multiplied by zero = 0, so (75)(0) = 0. Therefore x = 75 and y = 0; 75 > 0, so x > y.

56. C: If x = 3, then x2 = 9. To square a number, multiply it by itself. If x = 3 and x2 = 9, then x2 + x = 9 + 3 = 12.

57. B: If a = 4, then a2 = 16. The square of a number is that number multiplied by itself. You always perform the operation in parentheses first. So a2 + b = 16 + 5 = 21. Multiply 21 by 4 (the value of a). 21 * 4 = 84.

58. C: When adding and subtracting fractions, first you must find a common denominator. In this problem, there are fourths, halves, and thirds. Three does not divide evenly into 8, and 4 does not divide evenly into 6. But 4 * 3 = 12, and 12 is evenly divisible by 2, so use 12ths. Divide each denominator into 12, then multiply that quotient by each numerator: 1/4 = 3/12; 1/2 = 6/12; and 2/3 = 8/12. To solve this problem, respectively add and subtract the numerators: 3/12 + 6/12 = 9/12; 9/12 – 8/12 = 1/12, so the answer is 1/12.

59. B: To get a common denominator for /2, /3, and /8, multiply /8 * /3 = /24. Then 1/2 = 12/24; 1/3 = 8/24, and 3/8 = 9/24. The first operation is the one in

parentheses. If y = 8/24 and z = 9/24, y – z = 8/24 – 9/24. 8 – 9 yields a negative number, -1, or -1/24. If x = 12/24, then x * -1/24 = 12 * -1 in the numerator, or -12, and 24 * 24 in the denominator, or 576, giving -12/576. To reduce this fraction to the lowest possible numerator and denominator, divide each by 12. So -12/576 = -1/48.

60. D: To compare these two quantities, you need a common denominator. Multiply the first denominator, the 3 in 2/3, times the second denominator, the 4 in 1/4. 3 * 4 = 12. Divide the first original denominator into the common denominator, i.e., 12 ÷ 3 = 4, and multiply 4 * 2, the first numerator. 4 * 2 = 8. So 2/3 = 8/12. Do the same with the second fraction: 1/4 = 3/12. So if you have 3/12 cup of oil and you need a total of 8/12 cup, you need 5/12 cup more.

61. B: The common denominator for /4 and /2 = 4 * 2, or 8. Divide each fraction's denominator into the common denominator and multiply that quotient by each fraction's numerator. So 3/4 = 6/8, and 1/2 = 4/8. 6/8 + 4/8 = 10/8. 8 divides into 10 once, so 8/8 = 1 with 2/8 left over, making 1 and 2/8 or, reduced, 1¼. Add the whole numbers: 8 + 6 = 14. Then 14 + 1¼ = 15¼ .

62. D: If the first 10 minutes of the call cost $3.50 and the total charge was $3.85, just subtract $3.50 from $3.85 and you get $.35. Each additional minute cost $.35. So the call was 10 minutes plus 1 additional minute, for a total of 11 minutes.

63. A: If ½ cup of skim milk has 45 calories, then 1 cup has 90 calories (45 * 2 = 90, or 45 + 45 = 90). So ¼ cup is 90 calories ÷ 4 = 22.5 calories. For ¾, multiply 22.5 calories times 3 = 67.5 calories, that is, 67½. Another way to solve this is: ¼ = 25% or .25, so ¾ = 75% or .75. Multiply 90 * .75 = 67.5.

64. D: If a = 3, then 5a = 5 * 3 = 15. If 5a = 15, then 5a – 15 = 15 – 15 = 0. Because any number multiplied by 0 = 0, if 10b = 0, then b must also = 0.

65. C: Always perform the operations within the parentheses first before performing the operation between the parenthetical values. In this problem, 5 * 4 = 20 and 2 * 2 = 4. So 20 ÷ 4 = 5.

66. D: A prime number is any natural number that can only be divided evenly by 1 or by itself and not by any other numbers. For example, 2, 3, 5, 7, 11, 13, 17, and 19 are the first eight prime numbers in ascending order. Therefore, out of the choices given, 11 is the only prime number. 12 can be evenly divided by 2, 3, 4, and 6; 4 is evenly divisible by 2; and 15 is evenly divisible by 3 and 5. Furthermore, they are all evenly divisible by 1 and by themselves, so they are not prime numbers.

67. B: From the total of 23 club members, subtract the 12 females. 23 – 12 = 11, so there are 11 male members. To get the percentage of males, 11 ÷ 23 =0.478, which

rounds up to 0.48, or 48%. You can always get a percentage by dividing the smaller number by the larger number.

68. A: To obtain the percentage, divide the smaller number by the larger number. So $14 \div 57 = 0.245$, which rounds up to 0.25, or 25%. (Always round up when the next decimal place > 5.)

69. B: One simple way to figure this out is: 60% = 6/10. So if 75 = 6/10, find out how much 1/10 is: $75 \div 6 = 12.5$. So 12.5 = 1/10 of the unknown number. To get that number, just multiply the 1/10 by 10: $12.5 * 10 = 125$. With decimal numbers, you simply move the decimal point one place to the right instead, which is the same as multiplying by 10.

70. A: If the student receives $400.00 over 4 years, the average amount is $100.00 per year. ($400 ÷ 4 = $100.) Percentages can be calculated by dividing the smaller number by the bigger number. So to find out what percent $100.00 is of $3,000.00: $100 \div 3,000 = 0.033$, or 3.3%, which is the average annual interest rate.

Science Review

71. C: The heart's four chambers are the left and right atria, and the left and right ventricles. The left atrium and right atrium each hold blood returning to the heart via blood vessels, and each empties into the corresponding left or right ventricle at the right time. The ventricles are muscular and pump blood out of the heart. The right ventricle pumps blood to the lungs, and the left ventricle pumps blood to all the other organs.

72. A: Blood leaves the heart's right ventricle and goes to the lungs. The kidneys and the rest of the body receive blood from the left ventricle. The right atrium, as well as the left atrium, holds blood coming to the heart via the blood vessels; each atrium empties into the corresponding ventricle.

73. D: Anaerobic cellular metabolism refers to processes of breaking things down and converting them to other substances (metabolites) in the body's cells. Anaerobic means these processes do not use or require oxygen. Metabolic processes not involving oxygen do not affect heart rate. Increases in body temperature and physical activity increase the heart rate as the heart works harder to pump blood-supplying oxygen to the body. The concentrations of calcium, sodium, and potassium ions do affect heart rate. These ions, known as electrolytes, must stay in balance to regulate heart rate. If they are balanced, heart function is not affected, but with imbalance, cardiac function will be elevated (excess calcium) or depressed (excess potassium or sodium). Sodium deficiency causes cardiac fibrillation.

74. D: The three layers of the heart are the epicardium (outermost), myocardium (middle), and endocardium (innermost). "Vasocardium" is not a layer of the heart or even a legitimate term. The adjectives "vasocardial" or "vasocardiac" are used to

refer to anything related to both blood vessels (vaso-) and heart (cardiac), as with the "vasocardial system." A related term with the order of parts reversed is "cardiovascular system."

75. C: The hormone aldosterone is secreted by the adrenal glands and regulates the levels of sodium and potassium ions (electrolytes). Aldosterone stimulates excretion of potassium and reabsorption of sodium into the bloodstream. It maintains blood pressure and body fluids. Too much aldosterone can increase the blood volume and hence the blood pressure. Estrogen is a hormone of the female reproductive system and testosterone is a hormone of the male reproductive system. Dopamine is a neurotransmitter associated with the brain's pleasure and reward circuits, and also with the regulation of motor control.

76. B: Bradycardia means a slower heartbeat than normal. The combining form brady- is from the Greek bradys meaning slow. Tachycardia means a faster heartbeat than normal. (Tachy- from Greek tachos means speed, as also in "tachometer.") Fibrillation means uncoordinated, ineffectual heart movements. A myocardial infarct is a type of heart attack.

77. A: Hematocrit is the red blood cell portion of the blood. Plasma is mainly water, plus some plasma proteins, blood glucose, and so on. Normal levels of hematocrit are around 36% to 45% for women, and about 40% to 50% for men. Thus, an approximate normal level is around 45%. A hematocrit >50% can cause blood clots and heart attacks with exertion. If a hematocrit is 45%, it follows that the remaining plasma portion of the blood would be 55%.

78. B: The slightly bigger right lung has three lobes: the superior lobe, middle lobe, and inferior lobe. The left lung has two lobes: the superior lobe and the inferior lobe. So 3, 2 is the correct answer.

79. C: The aerobic respiration process has four steps. The first step, glycolysis, occurs in the cytoplasm. The second through fourth steps (the formation of acetyl coenzyme A, the citric acid cycle, and the electric transport chain and chemosmosis) occur in the mitochondria. Mitochondria are the cells' power producers. They create energy for cellular functions and processes, such as aerobic respiration, which involves the oxidation of glucose molecules.

80. B: Atelectasis is the medical term for collapse of a lung. Its Greek roots are ateles, incomplete or defective, and ektasis, extension or stretching out, as a collapsed lung cannot inflate and expand properly. Anoxia literally means no oxygen. It commonly refers to a lack of oxygen to the brain, especially in a fetus before or during childbirth. Dyspnea means difficulty breathing. Hypercapnia means too much carbon dioxide (a waste product of aerobic respiration) in the blood.

81. A: The central nervous system is another term for the brain and the spinal cord. It does not include the peripheral nerves (peripheral is the opposite of central) or the muscular system. Choices omitting the brain are necessarily incorrect.

82. C: The brain is composed of four lobes: the frontal lobe, the parietal lobe in the midbrain, the temporal lobe at the bottom, and the occipital lobe at the back. Some people also refer specifically to the left and right of each lobe. This is because the brain has two hemispheres (left and right), so each lobe also has two hemispheres. Each lobe has different functions.

83. C: Homeostasis is a state of equilibrium, or balance, within the body. The natural tendency is to maintain or restore homeostasis. Peristalsis is the wavelike muscular contractions of the digestive system to process food. Stomatitis is an inflammation of the mouth's mucosa.

84. D: Stomatitis is a state of oral inflammation, usually caused by viral or bacterial infection. Diverticulitis is inflammation of a diverticulum, or an abnormal pouch, in the wall of the large intestine. Hepatitis is inflammation of the liver. Enteritis is inflammation of the small intestine.

85. D: The most important male hormone is testosterone. Estrogen is the most important female hormone. Aldosterone is a hormone that regulates blood volume and pressure in both sexes. Progesterone is the second most important female hormone.

86. B: Bile production is a function of the liver, not of the kidneys. The kidneys filter the blood to clean it, removing waste products like urea and ammonium, excreting them in urine. They secrete hormones such as renin, calcitriol, and erythropoietin. The kidneys also reabsorb water, glucose, and amino acids.

87. A: Enuresis is the medical term for uncontrolled urination. A diuretic is an agent (a drug or substance) that stimulates urination. (Diuretics are not the same as enuresis but can cause it.) Pyuria means pus in the urine. Ureteritis means an inflammation of the ureter(s), muscular tubes that send urine from the kidneys into the bladder.

88. C: Auditory impulses, meaning sounds received through the ears, are interpreted in the brain's temporal lobes. Acoustic impulses travel through the external ear canal, are amplified and transmitted by the middle ear mechanism, converted into electrical energy in the inner ear's cochlea, and sent via the auditory nerve to the primary auditory cortex in the temporal lobe for analysis.

89. B: The eye's outer layer is the sclera, or the white of the eye. The cornea is the clear, protuberant, main refractive surface at the eye's front. The retina is a layered sensory tissue lining the eye's inner surface that is sensitive to light that creates

images of what the eye sees. The retina contains two kinds of photoreceptors: rods and cones. Cones are responsible for color vision and high visual acuity. Rods are responsible for peripheral vision, night vision/low-light vision, and detecting motion.

90. C: The inner layer of the eye is the retina. The cornea is the main refractive surface on the front of the eye. The sclera is the outermost layer, or white of the eye. The rods are one of two kinds of photoreceptors found within the retina. (The other photoreceptors are cones.)

91. D: Halogens are nonmetallic chemical elements. There are five halogens: fluorine, chlorine, bromine, iodine, and astatine. At room temperature, iodine and astatine are solids, bromine is a liquid, and fluorine and chlorine are gases. Cesium is not a halogen; it is a metal element.

92. A: In the periodic table of the chemical elements, the numbers of the periods 1, 2, 3, and so forth, are listed vertically in a column on the left, and each period runs horizontally across the table. The groups 1, 2, 3, et cetera, are listed horizontally, and each group runs vertically down the table.

93. A: The simplest unit of an element is an atom, i.e. the smallest particle to which it can be broken down. A molecule contains at least two atoms bonded together chemically (covalent bonding). Electrons, along with protons and neutrons, are particles found within the nucleus of an atom.

94. B: Isomers are compounds with the same shapes even if their structures vary. Polar compounds are molecules with polar covalent bonds; electromagnetically, their electrons are not equally shared in chemical bonds. Variables in the sciences are any entities or factors that can change. Experimenters manipulate variables to determine their effects on other variables. In research, a variable can be a logical set of attributes. A transient compound is one that disappears rapidly in the body.

95. C: Condensation is the process whereby gas is converted to liquid. For example, when water vapor (a gas) in the air is cooled, it becomes liquid. This is how condensation forms on the outside of a glass containing cold liquid. Evaporation is the opposite: the process of a liquid becoming a gas, as when water evaporates into the air. Sublimation is the process of a solid becoming a gas, as with dry ice.

96. B: Charles' Law is also known as the law of volumes. It describes how gases expand when heated. Boyle's law states that for a given mass at a constant temperature, the product of pressure times volume is a constant. Johnson's Law, attributed to California Senator Hiram Johnson (1918), states that "the first casualty when war comes is truth." Dr. Samuel Johnson (1730) had stated the same principle in much wordier terms. Avogadro's Law states that when a gas is at a constant

temperature and pressure, its volume is in direct proportion to the number of moles of gas. These are all gas laws except Johnson's.

97. A: The First Law of Thermodynamics states that neither matter nor energy can be created or destroyed. They can only be converted from one form to the other. Therefore, matter and energy are always conserved. The Second Law of Thermodynamics is the law of entropy: Energy moves away from its source, which means energy, or heat, cannot flow from a colder to a hotter body. The Third Law of Thermodynamics states that all energy processes cease as temperature approaches absolute zero. There is a "Zeroth" Law of Thermodynamics (if each of two systems is in equilibrium with a third system, the first two are in equilibrium with each other), but there is no "Fourth Law of Thermodynamics."

98. C: Acids increase the number of hydrogen ions in water. The pH scale measures how acidic or basic a liquid is. Hydrogen ions and hydroxide ions are the focus of pH. The strongest acids have low pH values: 0–4. High pH values (10–14) are found in the strongest bases or alkali, the opposites of acids. Sodium hydroxide is a base or alkaline compound. When dissolved in water, acids break down to hydrogen (H+) ions and another compound, while bases break down to hydroxide (OH-) ions and another compound.

99. D: A catalyst is a substance that increases the rate of a reaction. A reaction will not occur without the minimum activation energy it needs. A catalyst can provide an alternative means for the reaction to occur that requires a lower level of activation energy, so in this sense, a catalyst can also initiate a reaction. Another property of catalysts is that they do not change chemically after a reaction has completed, so they are never destroyed. Catalysts are not always on the right of the equation. For example, a car's catalytic converter takes harmful carbon monoxide and nitrogen oxide molecules and converts them, using platinum, palladium, and rhodium, to more harmless carbon dioxide and nitrogen molecules:

$2CO + 2NO \ \ Pt/Pd/Rh \rightarrow 2CO_2 + N_2$

The catalysts platinum (Pt), palladium (Pd), and rhodium (Rh) are in the middle of the equation.

100. A: Newton's Second Law of Motion states that when all existing forces are not balanced, the acceleration of an object depends on the net force acting on the object and the object's mass. When net force is represented as Fnet and mass as m, and acceleration as a, net force is the product of mass times acceleration, or F net = ma (or m * a). Speed = Distance/Time is the equation of the basic formula for calculating velocity. Power = F * D/T is the basic equation for work done, that is, force times distance divided by time. The formula of voltage times amperes is for calculating watts, or units of power, in the measurement of electrical energy.

Special Report: Nursing Exam Secrets in Action

Sample Question from the Mathematics Test:

Three coins are tossed up in the air. What is the probability that two of them will land heads and one will land tails?

A. 0
B. 1/8
C. 1/4
D. 3/8

Let's look at a few different methods and steps to solving this problem.

1. Reduction and Division

Quickly eliminate the probabilities that you immediately know. You know to roll all heads is a 1/8 probability, and to roll all tails is a 1/8 probability. Since there are in total 8/8 probabilities, you can subtract those two out, leaving you with 8/8 – 1/8 – 1/8 = 6/8. So after eliminating the possibilities of getting all heads or all tails, you're left with 6/8 probability. Because there are only three coins, all other combinations are going to involve one of either head or tail, and two of the other. All other combinations will either be 2 heads and 1 tail, or 2 tails and 1 head. Those remaining combinations both have the same chance of occurring, meaning that you can just cut the remaining 6/8 probability in half, leaving you with a 3/8ths chance that there will be 2 heads and 1 tail, and another 3/8ths chance that there will be 2 tails and 1 head, making choice D correct.

2. Run Through the Possibilities for that Outcome

You know that you have to have two heads and one tail for the three coins. There are only so many combinations, so quickly run through them all.

You could have:
H, H, H
H, H, T
H, T, H
T, H, H
T, T, H
T, H, T
H, T, T
T, T, T

Reviewing these choices, you can see that three of the eight have two heads and one tail, making choice D correct.

3. Fill in the Blanks with Symbology and Odds

Many probability problems can be solved by drawing blanks on a piece of scratch paper (or making mental notes) for each object used in the problem, then filling in probabilities and multiplying them out. In this case, since there are three coins being flipped, draw three blanks. In the first blank, put an "H" and over it write "1/2". This represents the case where the first coin is flipped as heads. In that case (where the first coin comes up heads), one of the other two coins must come up tails and one must come up heads to fulfill the criteria posed in the problem (2 heads and 1 tail). In the second blank, put a "1" or "1/1". This is because it doesn't matter what is flipped for the second coin, so long as the first coin is heads. In the third blank, put a "1/2". This is because the third coin must be the exact opposite of whatever is in the second blank. Half the time the third coin will be the same as the second coin, and half the time the third coin will be the opposite, hence the "1/2". Now multiply out the odds. There is a half chance that the first coin will come up "heads", then it doesn't matter for the second coin, then there is a half chance that the third coin will be the opposite of the second coin, which will give the desired result of 2 heads and 1 tail. So, that gives 1/2*1/1*1/2 = 1/4.

But, now you must calculate the probabilities that result if the first coin is flipped tails. So draw another group of three blanks. In the first blank, put a "T" and over it write "1/2". This represents the case where the first coin is flipped as tails. In that case (where the first coin comes up tails), both of the other two coins must come up heads to fulfill the criteria posed in the problem. In the second blank, put an "H" and over it write "1/2". In the third blank, put an "H" and over it write "1/2". Now multiply out the odds. There is a half chance that the first coin will come up "tails", then there is a half chance that the second coin will be heads, and a half chance that the third coin will be heads. So, that gives 1/2*1/2*1/2 = 1/8.

Now, add those two probabilities together. If you flip heads with the first coin, there is a 1/4 chance of ultimately meeting the problem's criteria. If you flip tails with the first coin, there is a 1/8 chance of ultimately meeting the problem's criteria. So, that gives 1/4 + 1/8 = 2/8 + 1/8 = 3/8, which makes choice D correct.

Sample Question from the Verbal Test:

Mark Twain was well aware of his celebrity. He was among the first authors to employ a clipping service to track press coverage of himself, and it was not unusual for him to issue his own press statements if he wanted to influence or "spin" coverage of a particular story. The celebrity Twain achieved during his last ten years still reverberates today. Nearly all of his most popular novels were published before 1890, long before his hair grayed or he began to wear his famous white suit in public. We appreciate the author but seem to remember the celebrity.

Based on the passage above, Mark Twain seemed interested in:

   A. maintaining his celebrity
   B. selling more of his books
   C. hiding his private life
   D. gaining popularity

Let's look at a couple of different methods of solving this problem.

1. Identify the key words in each answer choice. These are the nouns and verbs that are the most important words in the answer choice.

A. maintaining, celebrity
B. selling, books
C. hiding, life
D. gaining, popularity

Now try to match up each of the key words with the passage and see where they fit. You're trying to find synonyms and/or exact replication between the key words in the answer choices and key words in the passage.
A. maintaining – no matches; celebrity – matches in sentences 1, 3, and 5
B. selling – no matches; books – matches with "novels" in sentence 4.
C. hiding – no matches; life – no matches
D. gaining – no matches; popularity –matches with "celebrity" in sentences 1, 3, and
   5, because they can be synonyms

At this point there are only two choices that have more than one match, choices A and D, and they both have the same number of matches, and with the same word in the passage, which is the word "celebrity" in the passage. This is a good sign, because the test writers will often write two answer choices that are close. Having two answer choices pointing towards the same key word is a strong indicator that those key words hold the "key" to finding the right answer.

Now let's compare choice A and D and the unmatched key words. Choice A still has "maintaining" which doesn't have a clear match, while choice D has "gaining" which doesn't have a clear match. While neither of those have clear matches in the passage, ask yourself what are the best arguments that would support any kind of connection with either of those two words.

"Maintaining" makes sense when you consider that Twain was interested in tracking his press coverage and that he was actively managing the "spin" of certain stories.

"Gaining" makes sense when you consider that Twain was actively issuing his own press releases, however one key point to remember is that he was only issuing these press releases after another story was already in existence.

Since Twain's press releases were not being released in a news vacuum, but rather as a response mechanism to ensure control over the angle of a story, his releases were more to *maintain* control over his image, rather than *gain* an image in the first place.
Furthermore, when comparing the terms "popularity" and "celebrity", there are similarities between the words, but in referring back to the passage, it is clear that "celebrity" has a stronger connection to the passage, being the exact word used three times in the passage.

Since "celebrity" has a stronger match than "popularity" and "maintaining" makes more sense than "gaining," it is clear that choice A is correct.

2. Use a process of elimination.

A. maintaining his celebrity – The passage discusses how Mark Twain was both aware of his celebrity status and would take steps to ensure that he got the proper coverage in any news story and maintained the image he desired. This is the correct answer.

B. selling more of his books – Mark Twain's novels are mentioned for their popularity and while common sense would dictate that he would be interested in selling more of his books, the passage makes no mention of him doing anything to promote sales.

C. hiding his private life – While the passage demonstrates that Mark Twain was keenly interested in how the public viewed his life, it does not indicate that he cared about hiding his private life, not even mentioning his life outside of the public eye. The passage deals with how he was seen by the public.

D. gaining popularity – At first, this sounds like a good answer choice, because Mark Twain's popularity is mentioned several times. The main difference though is that he wasn't trying to gain popularity, but simply ensuring that the popularity he had was not distorted by bad press.

Sample Question from the Science Test:

Table 1

Length of 0.10 mm diameter aluminum wire (m)	Resistance (ohms) at 20° C
1	3.55
2	7.10
4	14.20
10	35.50

Based on the information in Table 1, one would predict that a 20 m length of aluminum wire with a 0.10 mm diameter would have a resistance of:

A. 16 ohms
B. 25 ohms
C. 34 ohms
D. 71 ohms

Let's look at a few different methods and steps to solving this problem.

1. Create a Proportion or Ratio

The first way you could approach this problem is by setting up a proportion or ratio. You will find that many of the problems on the RN Pre-entrance exam can be solved using this simple technique. Usually whenever you have a given pair of numbers (this number goes with that number) and you are given a third number and asked to find what number would be its match, then you have a problem that can be converted into an easy proportion or ratio.

In this case you can take any of the pairs of numbers from Table 1. As an example, let's choose the second set of numbers (2 m and 7.10 ohms).

Form a question with the information you have at your disposal: 2 meters goes to 7.10 ohms as 20 meters (from the question) goes to which resistance?

From your ratio: 2m/7.10 ohms = 20m/x
"x" is used as the missing number that you will solve for.

Cross multiplication provides us with 2*x = 7.10*20 or 2x = 142.

Dividing both sides by 2 gives us 2x/2 = 142/2 or x = 71, making choice D correct.

2. Use Algebra

The question is asking for the resistance of a 20 m length of wire. The resistance is a function of the length of the wire, so you know that you could probably set up an algebra problem that would have 20 multiplied by some factor "x" that would give you your answer.

So, now you have 20*x = ?

But what exactly is "x"? If 20*x would give you the resistance of a 20 foot piece of wire, than 1*x would give you the resistance of a 1 foot piece of wire. Remember though, the table already told you the resistance of a 1 foot piece of wire – it's 3.55 ohms.

So, if 1*x = 3.55 ohms, then solving for "x" gives you x = 3.55 ohms.

Plugging your solution for "x" back into your initial equation of 20*x = ?, you now have 20*3.55 ohms = 71 ohms, making choice D correct.

3. Look for a Pattern

Much of the time you can get by with just looking for patterns on problems that provide you with a lot of different numbers. In this case, consider the provided table.

        1 – 3.55
        2 – 7.10
        4 – 14.20
        10 – 35.50

What patterns do you see in the above number sequences. It appears that when the number in the first column doubled from 1 to 2, the numbers in the second column doubled as well, going from 3.55 to 7.10. Further inspection shows that when the numbers in the first column doubled from 2 to 4, the numbers in the second column doubled again, going from 7.10 to 14.20. Now you've got a pattern, when the first column of numbers doubles, so does the second column.

Since the question asked about a resistance of 20, you should recognize that 20 is the double of 10. Since a length of 10 meant a resistance of 35.50 ohms, then doubling the length of 10 should double the resistance, making 71 ohms, or choice D, correct.

4. Use Logic

A method that works even faster than finding patterns or setting up equations is using simple logic. It appears that as the first number (the length of the wire) gets larger, so does the second number (the resistance).

Since the length of 10 (the largest length wire in the provided table) has a corresponding resistance of 35.50, then another length (such as 20 in the question) should have a length greater than 35.50. As you inspect the answer choices, there is only one answer choice that is greater than 35.50, which is choice D, making it correct.

Secret Key #1 – Time is Your Greatest Enemy

To succeed on the RN Pre-entrance exam, you must use your time wisely. Most students do not finish at least one section.

The time constraints are brutal. To succeed, you must ration your time properly. The reason that time is so critical is that every question counts the same toward your final score. If you run out of time on any section, the questions that you do not answer will hurt your score far more than earlier questions that you spent extra time on and feel certain are correct.

Success Strategy #1

Pace Yourself

Wear a watch to the RN Pre-entrance exam. At the beginning of the test, check the time (or start a chronometer on your watch to count the minutes), and check the time after each passage or every few questions to make sure you are "on schedule."

If you find that you are falling behind time during the test, you must speed up. Even though a rushed answer is more likely to be incorrect, it is better to miss a couple of questions by being rushed, than to completely miss later questions by not having enough time. It is better to end with more time than you need than to run out of time.

If you are forced to speed up, do it efficiently. Usually one or more answer choices can be eliminated without too much difficulty. Above all, don't panic. Don't speed up and just begin guessing at random choices. By pacing yourself, and continually monitoring your progress against your watch, you will always know exactly how far ahead or behind you are with your available time. If you find that you are a few minutes behind on a section, don't skip questions without spending any time on it, just to catch back up. Begin spending a little less time per question and after a few questions, you will have caught back up more gradually. Once you catch back up, you can continue working each problem at your normal pace. If you have time at the end, go back then and finish the questions that you left behind.

Furthermore, don't dwell on the problems that you were rushed on. If a problem was taking up too much time and you made a hurried guess, it must have been difficult. The difficult questions are the ones you are most likely to miss anyway, so it isn't a big loss.

Last minute guessing will be covered in the next chapter.

Lastly, sometimes it is beneficial to slow down if you are constantly getting ahead of time. You are always more likely to catch a careless mistake by working more slowly than quickly, and among very high-scoring students (those who are likely to have lots of time left over), careless errors affect the score more than mastery of material.

Scanning

Don't waste time reading, enjoying, and completely understanding the passage. Simply scan the passage to get a rough idea of what it is about. You will return to the passage for each question, so there is no need to memorize it. Only spend as much time scanning as is necessary to get a vague impression of its overall subject content.

Secret Key #2 – Guessing is not guesswork.

Most students do not understand the impact that proper guessing can have on their score. Unless you score extremely high, guessing will contribute a significant amount of points to your score.

Monkeys Take the RN Pre-entrance Exam

What most students don't realize is that to insure that random 25% chance, you have to guess randomly. If you put 20 monkeys in a room to take the RN Pre-entrance exam, assuming they answered once per question and behaved themselves, on average they would get 25% of the questions correct. Put 20 students in the room, and the average will be much lower among guessed questions. Why?

1. The RN Pre-entrance exam intentionally has deceptive answer choices that "look" right. A student has no idea about a question, so picks the "best looking" answer, which is often wrong. The monkey has no idea what looks good and what doesn't, so will consistently be lucky about 25% of the time.
2. Students will eliminate answer choices from the guessing pool based on a hunch or intuition. Simple but correct answers often get excluded, leaving a 0% chance of being correct. The monkey has no clue, and often gets lucky with the best choice.

This is why the process of elimination endorsed by most test courses is flawed and detrimental to your performance- students don't guess, they make an ignorant stab in the dark that is usually worse than random.

Success Strategy #2

Let me introduce one of the most valuable ideas of this course- the $5 challenge:

You only mark your "best guess" if you are willing to bet $5 on it.
You only eliminate choices from guessing if you are willing to bet $5 on it.

Why $5? Five dollars is an amount of money that is small yet not insignificant, and can really add up fast (20 questions could cost you $100). Likewise, each answer choice on one question of the RN Pre-entrance exam will have a small impact on your overall score, but it can really add up to a lot of points in the end.

The process of elimination IS valuable. The following shows your chance of guessing it right:

If you eliminate this many choices:	0	1	2	3
Chance of getting it correct	25%	33%	50%	100%

However, if you accidentally eliminate the right answer or go on a hunch for an incorrect answer, your chances drop dramatically: to 0%. By guessing among all the answer choices, you are GUARANTEED to have a shot at the right answer.

That's why the $5 test is so valuable- if you give up the advantage and safety of a pure guess, it had better be worth the risk.

What we still haven't covered is how to be sure that whatever guess you make is truly random. Here's the easiest way:

Always pick the first answer choice among those remaining.

Such a technique means that you have decided, **before you see a single test question**, exactly how you are going to guess- and since the order of choices tells you nothing about which one is correct, this guessing technique is perfectly random.

Let's try an example-

A student encounters the following problem on the Mathematics test:

What is the cosine of an angle in a right triangle that is 3 meters on the adjacent side, 5 meters on the hypotenuse, and 4 meters on the opposite side?

A. 1
B. 0.6
C. 0.8
D. 1.25

The student has a small idea about this question- he is pretty sure that cosine is opposite over hypotenuse, but he wouldn't bet $5 on it. He knows that cosine is "something" over hypotenuse, and since the hypotenuse is the largest number, he is willing to bet $5 on both choices A and D not being correct. So he is down to B and C. At this point, he guesses B, since B is the first choice remaining.

The student is correct by choosing B, since cosine is adjacent over hypotenuse. He only eliminated those choices he was willing to bet money on, AND he did not let his stale memories (often things not known definitely will get mixed up in the exact opposite arrangement in one's head) about the formula for cosine influence his guess. He blindly chose the first remaining choice, and was rewarded with the fruits of a random guess.

This section is not meant to scare you away from making educated guesses or eliminating choices- you just need to define when a choice is worth eliminating. The $5 test, along with a pre-defined random guessing strategy, is the best way to make sure you reap all of the benefits of guessing.

Specific Guessing Techniques

Similar Answer Choices
When you have two answer choices that are direct opposites, one of them is usually the correct answer.
Example:
A.) forward
B.) backward

These two answer choices are very similar and fall into the same family of answer choices. A family of answer choices is when two or three answer choices are very similar. Often two will be opposites and one may show an equality.
Example:
A.) excited
B.) overjoyed
C.) thrilled
D.) upset

Note how the first three choices are all related. They all ask describe a state of happiness. However, choice D is not in the same family of questions. Being upset is the direct opposite of happiness.

Summary of Guessing Techniques
1. Eliminate as many choices as you can by using the $5 test. Use the common guessing strategies to help in the elimination process, but only eliminate choices that pass the $5 test.
2. Among the remaining choices, only pick your "best guess" if it passes the $5 test.
3. Otherwise, guess randomly by picking the first remaining choice that was not eliminated.

Secret Key #3 – Practice Smarter, Not Harder

Many students delay the test preparation process because they dread the awful amounts of practice time they think necessary to succeed on the test. We have refined an effective method that will take you only a fraction of the time.

There are a number of "obstacles" in your way on the RN Pre-entrance exam. Among these are answering questions, finishing in time, and mastering test-taking strategies. All must be executed on the day of the test at peak performance, or your score will suffer. The RN Pre-entrance exam is a mental marathon that has a large impact on your future.

Just like a marathon runner, it is important to work your way up to the full challenge. So first you just worry about questions, and then time, and finally strategy:

Success Strategy #3

1. Find a good source for RN Pre-entrance exam practice tests. A special report at the end gives you a good source for these. You will need at least 3 practice tests.
2. If you are willing to make a larger time investment (or if you want to really "learn" the material, a time consuming but ultimately valuable endeavor), consider buying one of the better study guides on the market
3. Take a practice test with no time constraints, with all study helps "open book." Take your time with questions and focus on applying the strategies.
4. Take another test, this time with time constraints, with all study helps "open book."
5. Take a final practice test with no open material and time limits.

If you have time to take more practice tests, just repeat step 5. By gradually exposing yourself to the full rigors of the test environment, you will condition your mind to the stress of test day and maximize your success.

Secret Key #4 – Prepare, Don't Procrastinate

Let me state an obvious fact: if you take the RN Pre-entrance exam three times, you will get three different scores. This is due to the way you feel on test day, the level of preparedness you have, and, despite RN Pre-entrance exam's claims to the contrary, some tests WILL be easier for you than others.

Since your acceptance will largely depend on your score, you should maximize your chances of success. In order to maximize the likelihood of success, you've got to prepare in advance. This means taking practice tests and spending time learning the information and test taking strategies you will need to succeed.

Since you have to pay a registration fee each time you take the RN Pre-entrance exam, don't take it as a "practice" test. Feel free to take sample tests on your own, but when you go to take the RN Pre-entrance exam, be prepared, be focused, and do your best the first time!

Secret Key #5 – Test Yourself

Everyone knows that time is money. There is no need to spend too much of your time or too little of your time preparing for the RN Pre-entrance exam. You should only spend as much of your precious time preparing as is necessary for you to pass it.

Success Strategy #5

Once you have taken a practice test under real conditions of time constraints, then you will know if you are ready for the test or not.

If you have scored extremely high the first time that you take the practice test, then there is not much point in spending countless hours studying. You are already there.

Benchmark your abilities by retaking practice tests and seeing how much you have improved. Once you score high enough to get accepted into the school of your choice, then you are ready.

If you have scored well below where you need, then knuckle down and begin studying in earnest. Check your improvement regularly through the use of practice tests under real conditions. Above all, don't worry, panic, or give up. The key is perseverance!

Then, when you go to take the RN Pre-entrance exam, remain confident and remember how well you did on the practice tests. If you can score high enough on a practice test, then you can do the same on the real thing.

General Strategies

The most important thing you can do is to ignore your fears and jump into the test immediately- do not be overwhelmed by any strange-sounding terms. You have to jump into the test like jumping into a pool- all at once is the easiest way.

Make Predictions
As you read and understand the question, try to guess what the answer will be. Remember that several of the answer choices are wrong, and once you begin reading them, your mind will immediately become cluttered with answer choices designed to throw you off. Your mind is typically the most focused immediately after you have read the question and digested its contents. If you can, try to predict what the correct answer will be. You may be surprised at what you can predict.

Quickly scan the choices and see if your prediction is in the listed answer choices. If it is, then you can be quite confident that you have the right answer. It still won't hurt to check the other answer choices, but most of the time, you've got it!

Answer the Question
It may seem obvious to only pick answer choices that answer the question, but the test writers can create some excellent answer choices that are wrong. Don't pick an answer just because it sounds right, or you believe it to be true. It MUST answer the question. Once you've made your selection, always go back and check it against the question and make sure that you didn't misread the question, and the answer choice does answer the question posed.

Benchmark
After you read the first answer choice, decide if you think it sounds correct or not. If it doesn't, move on to the next answer choice. If it does, mentally mark that answer choice. This doesn't mean that you've definitely selected it as your answer choice, it just means that it's the best you've seen thus far. Go ahead and read the next choice. If the next choice is worse than the one you've already selected, keep going to the next answer choice. If the next choice is better than the choice you've already selected, mentally mark the new answer choice as your best guess.

The first answer choice that you select becomes your standard. Every other answer choice must be benchmarked against that standard. That choice is correct until proven otherwise by another answer choice beating it out. Once you've decided that no other answer choice seems as good, do one final check to ensure that your answer choice answers the question posed.

Valid Information
Don't discount any of the information provided in the question. Every piece of information may be necessary to determine the correct answer. None of the

information in the question is there to throw you off (while the answer choices will certainly have information to throw you off). If two seemingly unrelated topics are discussed, don't ignore either. You can be confident there is a relationship, or it wouldn't be included in the question, and you are probably going to have to determine what is that relationship to find the answer.

Avoid "Fact Traps"
Don't get distracted by a choice that is factually true. Your search is for the answer that answers the question. Stay focused and don't fall for an answer that is true but incorrect. Always go back to the question and make sure you're choosing an answer that actually answers the question and is not just a true statement. An answer can be factually correct, but it MUST answer the question asked. Additionally, two answers can both be seemingly correct, so be sure to read all of the answer choices, and make sure that you get the one that BEST answers the question.

Milk the Question
Some of the questions may throw you completely off. They might deal with a subject you have not been exposed to, or one that you haven't reviewed in years. While your lack of knowledge about the subject will be a hindrance, the question itself can give you many clues that will help you find the correct answer. Read the question carefully and look for clues. Watch particularly for adjectives and nouns describing difficult terms or words that you don't recognize. Regardless of if you completely understand a word or not, replacing it with a synonym either provided or one you more familiar with may help you to understand what the questions are asking. Rather than wracking your mind about specific detailed information concerning a difficult term or word, try to use mental substitutes that are easier to understand.

The Trap of Familiarity
Don't just choose a word because you recognize it. On difficult questions, you may not recognize a number of words in the answer choices. The test writers don't put "make-believe" words on the test; so don't think that just because you only recognize all the words in one answer choice means that answer choice must be correct. If you only recognize words in one answer choice, then focus on that one. Is it correct? Try your best to determine if it is correct. If it is, that is great, but if it doesn't, eliminate it. Each word and answer choice you eliminate increases your chances of getting the question correct, even if you then have to guess among the unfamiliar choices.

Eliminate Answers
Eliminate choices as soon as you realize they are wrong. But be careful! Make sure you consider all of the possible answer choices. Just because one appears right, doesn't mean that the next one won't be even better! The test writers will usually put more than one good answer choice for every question, so read all of them. Don't worry if you are stuck between two that seem right. By getting down to just two

remaining possible choices, your odds are now 50/50. Rather than wasting too much time, play the odds. You are guessing, but guessing wisely, because you've been able to knock out some of the answer choices that you know are wrong. If you are eliminating choices and realize that the last answer choice you are left with is also obviously wrong, don't panic. Start over and consider each choice again. There may easily be something that you missed the first time and will realize on the second pass.

Tough Questions

If you are stumped on a problem or it appears too hard or too difficult, don't waste time. Move on! Remember though, if you can quickly check for obviously incorrect answer choices, your chances of guessing correctly are greatly improved. Before you completely give up, at least try to knock out a couple of possible answers. Eliminate what you can and then guess at the remaining answer choices before moving on.

Brainstorm

If you get stuck on a difficult question, spend a few seconds quickly brainstorming. Run through the complete list of possible answer choices. Look at each choice and ask yourself, "Could this answer the question satisfactorily?" Go through each answer choice and consider it independently of the other. By systematically going through all possibilities, you may find something that you would otherwise overlook. Remember that when you get stuck, it's important to try to keep moving.

Read Carefully

Understand the problem. Read the question and answer choices carefully. Don't miss the question because you misread the terms. You have plenty of time to read each question thoroughly and make sure you understand what is being asked. Yet a happy medium must be attained, so don't waste too much time. You must read carefully, but efficiently.

Face Value

When in doubt, use common sense. Always accept the situation in the problem at face value. Don't read too much into it. These problems will not require you to make huge leaps of logic. The test writers aren't trying to throw you off with a cheap trick. If you have to go beyond creativity and make a leap of logic in order to have an answer choice answer the question, then you should look at the other answer choices. Don't overcomplicate the problem by creating theoretical relationships or explanations that will warp time or space. These are normal problems rooted in reality. It's just that the applicable relationship or explanation may not be readily apparent and you have to figure things out. Use your common sense to interpret anything that isn't clear.

Prefixes

If you're having trouble with a word in the question or answer choices, try dissecting it. Take advantage of every clue that the word might include. Prefixes and suffixes can be a huge help. Usually they allow you to determine a basic meaning. Pre- means before, post- means after, pro - is positive, de- is negative. From these prefixes and suffixes, you can get an idea of the general meaning of the word and try to put it into context. Beware though of any traps. Just because con is the opposite of pro, doesn't necessarily mean congress is the opposite of progress!

Hedge Phrases

Watch out for critical "hedge" phrases, such as likely, may, can, will often, sometimes, often, almost, mostly, usually, generally, rarely, sometimes. Question writers insert these hedge phrases to cover every possibility. Often an answer choice will be wrong simply because it leaves no room for exception. Avoid answer choices that have definitive words like "exactly," and "always".

Switchback Words

Stay alert for "switchbacks". These are the words and phrases frequently used to alert you to shifts in thought. The most common switchback word is "but". Others include although, however, nevertheless, on the other hand, even though, while, in spite of, despite, regardless of.

New Information

Correct answer choices will rarely have completely new information included. Answer choices typically are straightforward reflections of the material asked about and will directly relate to the question. If a new piece of information is included in an answer choice that doesn't even seem to relate to the topic being asked about, then that answer choice is likely incorrect. All of the information needed to answer the question is usually provided for you, and so you should not have to make guesses that are unsupported or choose answer choices that require unknown information that cannot be reasoned on its own.

Time Management

On technical questions, don't get lost on the technical terms. Don't spend too much time on any one question. If you don't know what a term means, then since you don't have a dictionary, odds are you aren't going to get much further. You should immediately recognize terms as whether or not you know them. If you don't, work with the other clues that you have, the other answer choices and terms provided, but don't waste too much time trying to figure out a difficult term.

Contextual Clues

Look for contextual clues. An answer can be right but not correct. The contextual clues will help you find the answer that is most right and is correct. Understand the context in which a phrase or statement is made. This will help you make important distinctions.

Don't Panic

Panicking will not answer any questions for you. Therefore, it isn't helpful. When you first see the question, if your mind goes blank, take a deep breath. Force yourself to mechanically go through the steps of solving the problem and using the strategies you've learned.

Pace Yourself

Don't get clock fever. It's easy to be overwhelmed when you're looking at a page full of questions, your mind is full of random thoughts and feeling confused, and the clock is ticking down faster than you would like. Calm down and maintain the pace that you have set for yourself. As long as you are on track by monitoring your pace, you are guaranteed to have enough time for yourself. When you get to the last few minutes of the test, it may seem like you won't have enough time left, but if you only have as many questions as you should have left at that point, then you're right on track!

Answer Selection

The best way to pick an answer choice is to eliminate all of those that are wrong, until only one is left and confirm that is the correct answer. Sometimes though, an answer choice may immediately look right. Be careful! Take a second to make sure that the other choices are not equally obvious. Don't make a hasty mistake. There are only two times that you should stop before checking other answers. First is when you are positive that the answer choice you have selected is correct. Second is when time is almost out and you have to make a quick guess!

Check Your Work

Since you will probably not know every term listed and the answer to every question, it is important that you get credit for the ones that you do know. Don't miss any questions through careless mistakes. If at all possible, try to take a second to look back over your answer selection and make sure you've selected the correct answer choice and haven't made a costly careless mistake (such as marking an answer choice that you didn't mean to mark). This quick double check should more than pay for itself in caught mistakes for the time it costs.

Beware of Directly Quoted Answers

Sometimes an answer choice will repeat word for word a portion of the question or reference section. However, beware of such exact duplication – it may be a trap! More than likely, the correct choice will paraphrase or summarize a point, rather than being exactly the same wording.

Slang

Scientific sounding answers are better than slang ones. An answer choice that begins "To compare the outcomes..." is much more likely to be correct than one that begins "Because some people insisted..."

Extreme Statements

Avoid wild answers that throw out highly controversial ideas that are proclaimed as established fact. An answer choice that states the "process should be used in certain situations, if..." is much more likely to be correct than one that states the "process should be discontinued completely." The first is a calm rational statement and doesn't even make a definitive, uncompromising stance, using a hedge word "if" to provide wiggle room, whereas the second choice is a radical idea and far more extreme.

Answer Choice Families

When you have two or more answer choices that are direct opposites or parallels, one of them is usually the correct answer. For instance, if one answer choice states "x increases" and another answer choice states "x decreases" or "y increases," then those two or three answer choices are very similar in construction and fall into the same family of answer choices. A family of answer choices is when two or three answer choices are very similar in construction, and yet often have a directly opposite meaning. Usually the correct answer choice will be in that family of answer choices. The "odd man out" or answer choice that doesn't seem to fit the parallel construction of the other answer choices is more likely to be incorrect.

Appendix: Area, Volume, Surface Area Formulas

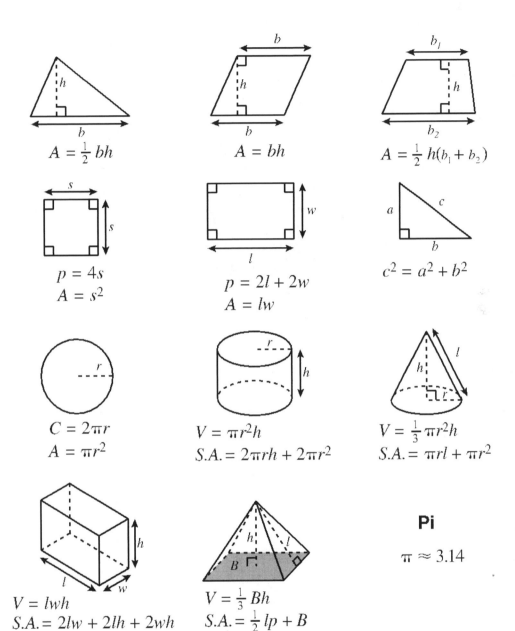

$A = \frac{1}{2}\,bh$

$A = bh$

$A = \frac{1}{2}\,h(b_1 + b_2)$

$p = 4s$
$A = s^2$

$p = 2l + 2w$
$A = lw$

$c^2 = a^2 + b^2$

$C = 2\pi r$
$A = \pi r^2$

$V = \pi r^2 h$
$S.A. = 2\pi rh + 2\pi r^2$

$V = \frac{1}{3}\,\pi r^2 h$
$S.A. = \pi rl + \pi r^2$

$V = lwh$
$S.A. = 2lw + 2lh + 2wh$

$V = \frac{1}{3}\,Bh$
$S.A. = \frac{1}{2}\,lp + B$

Pi

$\pi \approx 3.14$

Special Report: Musculature/Innervation Review of the Arm and Back

Muscle	Origin	Insertion	Nerve
Trapezius	Ext. Occipit Protuberance, Spines of T Vertebrae	Lateral Clavicle, Spine of the Scapula	Spinal Accessory Nerve CN XI
Latissimus Dorsi	Spines of Lower 6 T Vertebrae, Iliac Crest and Lower 4 Ribs	Bicipital Groove	Thoracodorsal
Levator Scapulae	Transverse Process of C1-C4	Upper Medial Border of Scapula	Dorsal Scapula
Rhomboid Major	Spinous Process of T2-T5	Medial Border Scapula Below Spine	Dorsal Scapular
Rhomboid Minor	Spinous Process of C7-T1	Medial Border Scapula Opp. Spine	Dorsal Scapular
Teres Major	Lateral Dorsal Inferior Angle of Scapula	Bicipital Groove	Lower Subscapular
Teres Minor	Lateral Scapula 2/3 way down	Greater Tubercle of Humerus	Axillary
Deltoid	Lateral 1/3 Clavicle and Acromion Process, Spine of the Scapula	Deltoid Tuberosity	Axillary
Supraspinatus	Supraspinatus Fossa	Greater Tubercle of Humerus	Suprascapular
Infraspinatus	Infaspinatus Fossa	Greater Tubercle of Humerus	Suprascapular
Subscapularis	Subscapular Fossa	Lesser Tubercle of Humerus	Upper and lower Subscapular
Serratus Anterior	Slips of Upper 8-9 Ribs	Ventral-Medial Border Scapula	Long Thoracic
Subclavius	Inferior Surface of the Clavicle	First Rib	Nerve to the Subclavius
Pectoralis Major	Medial ½ clavicle and Side of Sternum	Bicipital Groove	Medial and Lateral Pectoral
Pectoralis Minor	Ribs 3,4,5 or 2,3,4	Coracoid Process	Medial Pectoral
Biceps Branchii	Supraglenoid Tubercle	Posterior Margin of Radial Tuberosity	Musculocutaneous
Coracobrachialis	Coracoid Process	Medial Humerus at Deltoid Tuberosity Level	Musculocutaneous
Brachialis	Anterior-Lateral ½ of Humerus	Ulnar Tuberosity and Coronoid Process	Musculocutaneous
Triceps Brachii	Infraglenoid Tubercle, Below and Medial to the Radial Groove	Olecranon Process	Radial
Anconeus	Posterior, Lateral Humeral Condyle	Upper Posterior Ulna	Radial
Brachioradialis	Lateral Supracondylar Ridge of Humerus	Radial Styloid Process	Radial
Pronator Teres	Medial Epicondyle and Supracondylar Ridge	½ Way Down on Lateral Radius	Median
Pronator Quadratus	Distal-Medial Ulna	Distal-Lateral Radius	Anterior Interosseous

Musculature/Innervation Review of the Forearm

Muscle	Origin	Insertion	Nerve
Brachioradialis	Lateral Supracondylar Ridge of Humerus	Radial Styloid Process	Radial
Pronator Teres	Medial Epicondyle and Supracondylar Ridge	½ Way Down on Lateral Radius	Median
Pronator Quadratus	Distal-Medial Ulna	Distal-Lateral Radius	Anterior Interosseous
Supinator	Lateral Epicondyle of Humerus	Upper ½ Lateral, Posterior Radius	Posterior Inter-Deep Radial
Flexor Carpi Radialis	Medial Epicondyle of Humerus	2nd and 3rd Metacarpal	Median
Flexor Carpi Ulnaris	Medial Epicondyle of Humerus	Pisiform, Hamate, 5th Metacarpal	Ulnar
Palmaris Longus	Medial Epicondyle of the Humerus	Palmar Aponeurosis and Flexor Retinaculum	Median
Flexor Digitorum Suerficialis	Medial Epicondyle, Radius, Ulna	Medial 4 Digits	Median
Flexor Digitorum Profundus	Ulna, Interosseous Membrane	Medial 4 Digits (distal part)	Median (lateral 2 digits), Ulnar (median 2 digits)
Flexor Pollicis Longus	Radius	Distal Phalanx (thumb)	Anterior Inter-Deep Median
Extensor Carpi Radialis Longus	Lateral Condyle and Supracondylar Ridge	2nd Metacarpal	Radial
Extensor Carpi Radialis Brevis	Lateral Epicondyle of Humerus	3rd Metacarpal	Posterior Inter-Deep Radial
Extensor Carpi Ulnaris	Lateral Epicondyle of Humerus	5th Metacarpal	Posterior Inter-Deep Radial
Extensor Digitorum	Lateral Epicondyle of Humerus	Extension Expansion Hood of Medial 4 Digits	Posterior Inter-Deep Radial
Extensor Digiti Minimi	Lateral Epicondyle of Humerus	Extension Expansion Hood of (little finger)	Posterior Inter-Deep Radial
Abductor Pollicis Longus	Posterior Radius and Ulna	Radial Side of 1st Metacarpal	Posterior Inter-Deep Radial
Extensor Indicis	Ulna and Interosseous Membrane	Extension Expansion Hood (index finger)	Posterior Inter-Deep Radial
Extensor Pollicis Longus	Ulna and Interosseous Membrane	Distal Phalanx (thumb)	Posterior Inter-Deep Radial
Extensor Pollicis Brevis	Radius	Proximal Phalanx (thumb)	Posterior Inter-Deep Radial

Musculature/Innervation Review of the Hand

Muscle	Origin	Insertion	Nerve
Adductor Policis	Capitate and Base of Adjacent Metacarpals	Proximal Phalanx (thumb)	Deep Branch of Ulnar
Lumbricals	Tendons of Flexor Digitorum Profundas	Extension Expansion Hood of Medial 4 Digits	Deep Branch Ulnar (medial 2 Ls), Median (lateral 2 Ls)
Dorsal Interosseous Muscles (4)	Sides of Metacarpals	Extension Expansion Hood of Digits 2-4	Deep Branch Ulnar
Palmar Interosseous (3)	Sides of Metacarpals	Extension Expansion Hood, Digits 2,4,5	Deep Branch Ulnar
Palmaris Brevis	Anterior Flexor Retinaculum and Palmar Aponeurosis	Skin-Ulnar Border of Hand	Superficial Ulnar
Abductor Pollicis Brevis	Flexor Retinaculum, Trapezium	Lateral Proximal Phalanx (thumb)	Median (thenar branch)
Flexor Pollicis Brevis	Flexor Retinaculum, Trapezium	Lateral Proximal Phalanx (thumb)	Median (thenar branch)
Opponens Pollicis	Flexor Retinaculum, Trapezium	Radial Border (1st Metacarpal)	Median (thenar branch)
Abductor Digiti Minimi	Flexor Retinaculum, Pisiform	Proximal Phalanx (little finger)	Deep Branch Ulnar
Flexor Digiti Minimi	Flexor Retinaculum, Hamate	Proximal Phalanx (little finger)	Deep Branch Ulnar
Opponens Digiti Minimi	Flexor Retinaculum, Hamate	Ulnar Medial Border (5th Metacarpal)	Deep Branch Ulnar

Musculature/Innervation Review of the Thigh

Muscle	Origin	Insertion	Nerve
Psoas Major	Bodies and Discs of T12-L5	Lesser Trochanter	L2,3
Psoas Minor	Bodies and Discs of T12 and L1	Pectineal Line of Superior Pubic Bone	L2,3
Iliacus	Upper 2/3 Iliac Fossa	Lesser Trochanter	Femoral L2-4
Pectinius	Pubic Ramus	Spiral Line	Femoral
Iliposoas	Joining of Psoas Major and Iliacus	Lesser Trochanter	L2-4
Piriformis	Anterior Surface of the Sacrum	Greater Trochanter	S1, S2
Obturator Internus	Inner Surface of the Obturator Membrane	Greater Trochanter	Sacral Plexus
Obturator Externus	Outer Surface of the Obturator Membrane	Greater Trochanter	Obturator
Gemellus Superior	Ischial Spine	Greater Trochanter	Sacral Plexus
Gemellus Inferior	Ischial Tuberosity	Greater Trochanter	Sacral Plexus
Quadratus Femoris	Ischial Tuberosity	Quadrate Tubercle of the Femur	Sacral Plexus
Gluteus Maximus	Outer Surface of Ilium, Sacrum and Coccyx	Iliotibial Tract, Gluteal Tubercle of the Femur	Inferior Gluteal
Gluteus Minimus	Outer Surface of the Ilium	Greater Trochanter	Superior Gluteal
Gluteus Medius	Outer Surface of the Ilium	Greater Trochanter	Superior Gluteal
Satorius	Anterior Superior Iliac Spine	Upper Medial Tibia	Femoral
Quadriceps Femoris	Anterior Inferior Iliac Spine, Femur-Lateral and Medial	Tibial Tuberosity	Femoral
Gracilis	Pubic Bone	Upper Medial Tibia	Obturator (anterior branch)
Abductor Longus	Pubic Bone	Linea Aspera	Obturator (anterior branch)
Abductor Brevis	Pubic Bone	Linea Aspera	Obturator (anterior branch)
Abductor Magnus	Pubic Bone	Entire Linea Aspera	Sciatic, Obturator
Tensor Faciae Latae	Iliac Crest	Iliotibial Band	Superior Gluteal
Biceps Femoris	Ischial Tuberosity, Linea Aspera	Head of Fibula, Lateral Condyle of Tibia	Sciatic-Tibial portion and Common Peroneal Portion
Semimembranosus	Ischial Tuberosity	Upper Medial Tibia	Sciatic-Tibial Portion
Semitendinosus	Ischial Tuberosity	Upper Medial Tibia	Sciatic-Tibial Portion

Musculature/Innervation Review of the Calf and Foot

Muscle	Origin	Insertion	Nerve
Tibialis Anterior	Upper 2/3 Lateral Tibia and Interosseous Membrane	1st Cuneiform and Base of 1st Metatarsal	Deep Peroneal
Extensor Digitorum Longus	Upper 2/3 Fibula and Interosseous Membrane	4 Tendons-Distal Middle Phalanges	Deep Peroneal
Extensor Hallucis Longus	Middle 1/3 of Anterior Fibula	Base of Distal Phalanx of Big Toe	Deep Peroneal
Peroneus Tertius	Distal Fibula	Base of 5th Metatarsal	Deep Peroneal
Extensor Hallucis Brevis	Dorsal Calcaneus	Extensor Digitorum Longus Tendons	Deep Peroneal
Peroneus Longus	Upper 2/3 Lateral Fibula	1st Metatarsal and 1st Cuneiform	Superficial Peroneal
Peroneus Brevis	Lateral Distal Fibula	5th Metatarsal Tuberosity	Superficial Peroneal
Soleus	Upper Shaft of Fibula	Calcaneus via Achilles Tendon	Tibial
Flexor Digitorum Longus	Middle 1/3 of Posterior Tibia	Base of Distal Phalanx of Lateral 4 Toes	Tibial
Flexor Hallucis Longus	Middle and Lower 1/3 of Posterior Tibia	Distal Phalanx of Big Toe	Tibial
Tibialis Posterior	Posterior Upper Tibia, Fibula	Navicular Bone and 1st Cuneiform	Tibial
Popliteus	Upper Posterior Tibia	Lateral Condyle of Femur	Tibial
Flexor Digitorum Brevis	Calcaneus	Middle Phalanges of Lateral 4 Toes	Medial Plantar
Abductor Hallucis	Calcaneus	Medial Proximal Phalanx of Big Toe	Medial Plantar
Abductor Digiti Brevis	Calcaneus	Lateral Proximal Phalanx of Big Toe	Lateral Plantar
Quadratus Plantae	Lateral and Medial Side of the Calcaneus	Tendons of Flexor Digitorum Longus	Lateral Plantar
Lumbricals	Tendons of Flexor Digitorum Longus	Extensor Tendons of Toes	Medial Plantar/Lateral Plantar
Flexor Hallucis Brevis	Cuboid Bone	Splits on Base of Proximal Phalanx of Big Toe	Medial Plantar
Flexor Digiti Minimi Brevis	Base of 5th Metatarsal	Base of Proximal Phalanx of Little Toe	Lateral Plantar
Abductor Hallucis	Metatarsals 2-4	Base of Proximal Phalanx of Big Toe	Lateral Plantar
Interossei	Sides of Metatarsal Bones	Base of 1st Phalanx and Extensor Tendons	Lateral Plantar

CPR Review/Cheat Sheet

Topic	New Guidelines
Conscious Choking	5 back blows, then 5 abdominal thrusts- adult/child
Unconscious Choking	5 chest compressions, look, 2 breaths-adult/child/infant
Rescue Breaths	Normal Breath given over 1 second until chest rises
Chest Compressions to Ventilation Ratios (Single Rescuer)	30:2 – Adult/Child/Infant
Chest Compressions to Ventilation Ratios (Two Rescuer)	30:2 – Adult 15:2 – Child/Infant
Chest Compression rate	About 100/minute – Adult/Child/Infant
Chest Compression Land marking Method	Simplified approach – center of the chest – Adult/Child 2 or 3 fingers, just below the nipple line at the center of the chest - Infant
AED	1 shock, then 2 minutes (or 5 cycles) of CPR
Anaphylaxis	Assist person with use of prescribed auto injector
Asthma	Assist person with use of prescribed inhaler

- Check the scene
- Check for responsiveness – ask, "Are you OK?"
- Adult - call 911, then administer CPR
- Child/Infant – administer CPR for 5 cycles, then call 911
- Open victim's airway and check for breathing – look, listen, and feel for 5 - 10 seconds
- Two rescue breaths should be given, 1 second each, and should produce a visible chest rise
- If the air does not go in, reposition and try 2 breaths again
- Check victim's pulse – chest compressions are recommended if an infant or child has a rate less than 60 per minute with signs of poor perfusion.
- Begin 30 compressions to 2 breaths at a rate of 1 breath every 5 seconds for Adult; 1 breath every 3 seconds for child/infant
- Continue 30:2 ratio until victim moves, AED is brought to the scene, or professional help arrives

AED
- ADULT/ Child over 8 years old - use Adult pads
- Child 1-8 years old – use Child pads or use Adult pads by placing one on the chest and one on the back of the child
- Infant under 1 year of age - AED not recommended

Special Report: Pharmacology Generic/Trade Names of 50 Key Drugs in Medicine

1. Alprazolam	XANAX
2. Amitriptyline	ELAVIL
3. Amoxicillin/clavulanate potassium	AUGMENTIN
4. Betamethasone	CELESTONE
5. Bumetanide	BUMEX
6. Bupropion	WELLBUTRIN
7. Calcitriol	ROCALTROL
8. Ceforanide	PRECEF
9. Ceftazidime	FORTAZ
10. Cephalexin	KEFLEX
11. Ciprofloxacin	CIPRO
12. Clonazepam	KLONOPIN
13. Cyclobenzaprine	FLEXERIL
14. Diazepam	VALIUM
15. Dopamine	INTROPIN
16. Enalapril	VASOTEC
17. Eythromycin	E-MYCIN
18. Famotidine	PEPCID
19. Fluconazole	DiFLUCON
20. Fluoxetine	PROZAC
21. Furosemide	LASIX
22. Gentamicin	GARAMYCIN
23. Haloperidol	HALDOL
24. Hydroxyprogesterone caproate	DELALUTIN
25. Ibuprofen	MOTRIN
26. Ipratropium bromide	ATROVENT
27. Ketorolac	TORADOL
28. Lidocaine	XYLOCAINE
29. Lorazepam	ATIVAN
30. Meperidine	DEMEROL
31. Methicillin	STAPHCILLIN
32. Metoprolol	LOPRESSOR
33. Miconazole	MONISTAT
34. Nystatin	MYCOSTATIN
35. Omeprazole	PRILOSEC
36. Oxybutynin	DITROPAN
37. Oxymetholone	ANADROL
38. Pergolide	PERMAX
39. Phenytoin	DILANTIN
40. Prazepam	CENTRAX

41.	Prednisone	DELTASONE
42.	Procaine	NOVOCAIN
43.	Promethazine	PHENERGAN
44.	Propoxyphene	DARVON
45.	Pseudoephedrine	SUDAFED
46.	Silver sulfadiazine	SILVADENE
47.	Temazepam	RESTORIL
48.	Tolnaftate	TINACTIN
49.	Vancomycin	VANCOCIN
50.	Warfarin	COUMADIN

Special Report: How to Overcome Your Fear of Math

If this article started by saying "Math," many of us would feel a shiver crawl up our spines, just by reading that simple word. Images of torturous years in those crippling desks of the math classes can become so vivid to our consciousness that we can almost smell those musty textbooks, and see the smudges of the #2 pencils on our fingers.

If you are still a student, feeling the impact of these sometimes overwhelming classroom sensations, you are not alone if you get anxious at just the thought of taking that compulsory math course. Does your heart beat just that much faster when you have to split the bill for lunch among your friends with a group of your friends? Do you truly believe that you simply don't have the brain for math? Certainly you're good at other things, but math just simply isn't one of them? Have you ever avoided activities, or other school courses because they appear to involve mathematics, with which you're simply not comfortable?

If any one or more of these "symptoms" can be applied to you, you could very well be suffering from a very real condition called "Math Anxiety."

It's not at all uncommon for people to think that they have some sort of math disability or allergy, when in actuality, their block is a direct result of the way in which they were taught math!

In the late 1950's with the dawning of the space age, New Math - a new "fuzzy math" reform that focuses on higher-order thinking, conceptual understanding and solving problems - took the country by storm. It's now becoming ever more clear that teachers were not supplied with the correct, practical and effective way in which they should be teaching new math so that students will understand the methods comfortably. So is it any wonder that so many students struggled so deeply, when their teachers were required to change their entire math systems without the foundation of proper training? Even if you have not been personally, directly affected by that precise event, its impact is still as rampant as ever.

Basically, the math teachers of today are either the teachers who began teaching the new math in the first place (without proper training) or they are the students of the math teachers who taught new math without proper training. Therefore, unless they had a unique, exceptional teacher, their primary, consistent examples of teaching math have been teachers using methods that are not conducive to the general understanding of the entire class. This explains why your discomfort (or fear) of math is not at all rare.

It is very clear why being called up to the chalk board to solve a math problem is such a common example of a terrifying situation for students - and it has very little to do with a fear of being in front of the class. Most of us have had a minimum of one humiliating experience while standing with chalk dusted fingers, with the eyes of every math student piercing through us. These are the images that haunt us all the way through adulthood. But it does not mean that we cannot learn math. It just means that we could be developing a solid case of math anxiety.

But what exactly is math anxiety? It's an very strong emotional sensation of anxiety, panic, or fear that people feel when they think about or must apply their ability to understand mathematics. Sufferers of math anxiety frequently believe that they are incapable of doing activities or taking classes that involve math skills. In fact, some people with math anxiety have developed such a fear that it has become a phobia; aptly named math phobia.

The incidence of math anxiety, especially among college students, but also among high school students, has risen considerably over the last 10 years, and currently this increase shows no signs of slowing down. Frequently students will even chose their college majors and programs based specifically on how little math will be compulsory for the completion of the degree.

The prevalence of math anxiety has become so dramatic on college campuses that many of these schools have special counseling programs that are designed to assist math anxious students to deal with their discomfort and their math problems.

Math anxiety itself is not an intellectual problem, as many people have been lead to believe; it is, in fact, an emotional problem that stems from improper math teaching techniques that have slowly built and reinforced these feelings. However, math anxiety can result in an intellectual problem when its symptoms interfere with a person's ability to learn and understand math.

The fear of math can cause a sort of "glitch" in the brain that can cause an otherwise clever person to stumble over even the simplest of math problems. A study by Dr. Mark H. Ashcraft of Cleveland State University in Ohio showed that college students who usually perform well, but who suffer from math anxiety, will suffer from fleeting lapses in their working memory when they are asked to perform even the most basic mental arithmetic. These same issues regarding memory were not present in the same students when they were required to answer questions that did not involve numbers. This very clearly demonstrated that the memory phenomenon is quite specific to only math.

So what exactly is it that causes this inhibiting math anxiety? Unfortunately it is not as simple as one answer, since math anxiety doesn't have one specific cause. Frequently math anxiety can result of a student's either negative experience or embarrassment with math or a math teacher in previous years.

These circumstances can prompt the student to believe that he or she is somehow deficient in his or her math abilities. This belief will consistently lead to a poor performance in math tests and courses in general, leading only to confirm the beliefs of the student's inability. This particular phenomenon is referred to as the "self-fulfilling prophecy" by the psychological community. Math anxiety will result in poor performance, rather than it being the other way around.

Dr. Ashcraft stated that math anxiety is a "It's a learned, almost phobic, reaction to math," and that it is not only people prone to anxiety, fear, or panic who can develop math anxiety. The image alone of doing math problems can send the blood pressure and heart rate to race, even in the calmest person.

The study by Dr. Ashcraft and his colleague Elizabeth P. Kirk, discovered that students who suffered from math anxiety were frequently stumped by issues of even the most basic math rules, such as "carrying over" a number, when performing a sum, or "borrowing" from a number when doing a subtraction. Lapses such as this occurred only on working memory questions involving numbers.

To explain the problem with memory, Ashcraft states that when math anxiety begins to take its effect, the sufferer experiences a rush of thoughts, leaving little room for the focus required to perform even the simplest of math problems. He stated that "you're draining away the energy you need for solving the problem by worrying about it."

The outcome is a "vicious cycle," for students who are sufferers of math anxiety. As math anxiety is developed, the fear it promotes stands in the way of learning, leading to a decrease in self-confidence in the ability to perform even simple arithmetic.

A large portion of the problem lies in the ways in which math is taught to students today. In the US, students are frequently taught the rules of math, but rarely will they learn why a specific approach to a math problems work. Should students be provided with a foundation of "deeper understanding" of math, it may prevent the development of phobias.

Another study that was published in the Journal of Experimental Psychology by Dr. Jamie Campbell and Dr. Qilin Xue of the University of Saskatchewan in Saskatoon, Canada, reflected the same concepts. The researchers in this study looked at university students who were educated in Canada and China, discovering that the Chinese students could generally outperform the Canadian-educated students when it came to solving complex math problems involving procedural knowledge - the ability to know how to solve a math problem, instead of simply having ideas memorized.

A portion of this result seemed to be due to the use of calculators within both elementary and secondary schools; while Canadians frequently used them, the Chinese students did not.

However, calculators were not the only issue. Since Chinese-educated students also outperformed Canadian-educated students in complex math, it is suggested that cultural factors may also have an impact. However, the short-cut of using the calculator may hinder the development of the problem solving skills that are key to performing well in math.

Though it is critical that students develop such fine math skills, it is easier said than done. It would involve an overhaul of the training among all elementary and secondary educators, changing the education major in every college.

Math Myths

One problem that contributes to the progression of math anxiety, is the belief of many math myths. These erroneous math beliefs include the following:

Men are better in math than women - however, research has failed to demonstrate that there is any difference in math ability between the sexes. There is a single best way to solve a math problem - however, the majority of math problems can be solved in a number of different ways. By saying that there is only one way to solve a math problem, the thinking and creative skills of the student are held back.

Some people have a math mind, and others do not - in truth, the majority of people have much more potential for their math capabilities than they believe of themselves.

It is a bad thing to count by using your fingers - counting by using fingers has actually shown that an understanding of arithmetic has been established. People who are skilled in math can do problems quickly in their heads - in actuality, even math professors will review their example problems before they teach them in their classes.

The anxieties formed by these myths can frequently be perpetuated by a range of mind games that students seem to play with themselves. These math mind games include the following beliefs:

- 137 -

I don't perform math fast enough - actually everyone has a different rate at which he or she can learn. The speed of the solving of math problems is not important as long as the student can solve it.

I don't have the mind for math - this belief can inhibit a student's belief in him or herself, and will therefore interfere with the student's real ability to learn math.

I got the correct answer, but it was done the wrong way - there is no single best way to complete a math problem. By believing this, a student's creativity and overall understanding of math is hindered.

If I can get the correct answer, then it is too simple - students who suffer from math anxiety frequently belittle their own abilities when it comes to their math capabilities.

Math is unrelated to my "real" life - by freeing themselves of the fear of math, math anxiety sufferers are only limiting their choices and freedoms for the rest of their life.

Fortunately, there are many ways to help those who suffer from math anxiety. Since math anxiety is a learned, psychological response to doing or thinking about math, that interferes with the sufferer's ability to understand and perform math, it is not at all a reflection of the sufferer's true math sills and abilities.

Helpful Strategies

Many strategies and therapies have been developed to help students to overcome their math anxious responses. Some of these helpful strategies include the following:

Reviewing and learning basic arithmetic principles, techniques and methods. Frequently math anxiety is a result of the experience of many students with early negative situations, and these students have never truly developed a strong base in basic arithmetic, especially in the case of multiplication and fractions. Since math is a discipline that is built on an accumulative foundation, where the concepts are built upon gradually from simpler concepts, a student who has not achieved a solid basis in arithmetic will experience difficulty in learning higher order math. Taking a remedial math course, or a short math course that focuses on arithmetic can often make a considerable difference in reducing the anxious response that math anxiety sufferers have with math.

Becoming aware of any thoughts, actions and feelings that are related to math and responses to math. Math anxiety has a different effect on different students. Therefore it is very important to become familiar with any reactions that the

- 138 -

math anxiety sufferer may have about him/herself and the situation when math has been encountered. If the sufferer becomes aware of any irrational or unrealistic thoughts, it's possible to better concentrate on replacing these thoughts with more positive and realistic ones.

Find help! Math anxiety, as we've mentioned, is a learned response, that is reinforced repeatedly over a period of time, and is therefore not something that can be eliminated instantaneously. Students can more effectively reduce their anxious responses with the help of many different services that are readily available. Seeking the assistance of a psychologist or counselor, especially one with a specialty in math anxiety, can assist the sufferer in performing an analysis of his/her psychological response to math, as well as learning anxiety management skills, and developing effective coping strategies. Other great tools are tutors, classes that teach better abilities to take better notes in math class, and other math learning aids.

Learning the mathematic vocabulary will instantly provide a better chance for understanding new concepts. One major issue among students is the lack of understanding of the terms and vocabulary that are common jargon within math classes. Typically math classes will utilize words in a completely different way from the way in which they are utilized in all other subjects. Students easily mistake their lack of understanding the math terms with their mathematical abilities.

Learning anxiety reducing techniques and methods for anxiety management. Anxiety greatly interferes with a student's ability to concentrate, think clearly, pay attention, and remember new concepts. When these same students can learn to relax, using anxiety management techniques, the student can regain his or her ability to control his or her emotional and physical symptoms of anxiety that interfere with the capabilities of mental processing.

Working on creating a positive overall attitude about mathematics. Looking at math with a positive attitude will reduce anxiety through the building of a positive attitude.

Learning to self-talk in a positive way. Pep talking oneself through a positive self talk can greatly assist in overcoming beliefs in math myths or the mind games that may be played. Positive self-talking is an effective way to replace the negative thoughts - the ones that create the anxiety. Even if the sufferer doesn't believe the statements at first, it plants a positive seed in the subconscious, and allows a positive outlook to grow.

Beyond this, students should learn effective math class, note taking and studying techniques. Typically, the math anxious students will avoid asking questions to save themselves from embarrassment. They will sit in the back of classrooms, and refrain from seeking assistance from the professor. Moreover, they will put off studying for math until the very last moment, since it causes them such substantial discomfort. Alone, or a combination of these negative behaviors work only to reduce the anxiety of the students, but in reality, they are actually building a substantially more intense anxiety.

There are many different positive behaviors that can be adopted by math anxious students, so that they can learn to better perform within their math classes.

Sit near the front of the class. This way, there will be fewer distractions, and there will be more of a sensation of being a part of the topic of discussion. If any questions arise, ASK! If one student has a question, then there are certain to be others who have the same question but are too nervous to ask - perhaps because they have not yet learned how to deal with their own math anxiety.

Seek extra help from the professor after class or during office hours.

Prepare, prepare, prepare - read textbook material before the class, do the homework and work out any problems available within the textbook. Math skills are developed through practice and repetition, so the more practice and repetition, the better the math skills.

Review the material once again after class, to repeat it another time, and to reinforce the new concepts that were learned.

Beyond these tactics that can be taken by the students themselves, teachers and parents need to know that they can also have a large impact on the reduction of math anxiety within students.

As parents and teachers, there is a natural desire to help students to learn and understand how they will one day utilize different math techniques within their everyday lives. But when the student or teacher displays the symptoms of a person who has had nightmarish memories regarding math, where hesitations then develop in the instruction of students, these fears are automatically picked up by the students and commonly adopted as their own.

However, it is possible for teachers and parents to move beyond their own fears to better educate students by overcoming their own hesitations and learning to enjoy math.

Begin by adopting the outlook that math is a beautiful, imaginative or living thing. Of course, we normally think of mathematics as numbers that can be added or subtracted, multiplied or divided, but that is simply the beginning of it.

By thinking of math as something fun and imaginative, parents and teachers can teach children different ways to manipulate numbers, for example in balancing a checkbook. Parents rarely tell their children that math is everywhere around us; in nature, art, and even architecture. Usually, this is because they were never shown these relatively simple connections. But that pattern can break very simply through the participation of parents and teachers.

The beauty and hidden wonders of mathematics can easily be emphasized through a focus that can open the eyes of students to the incredible mathematical patterns that arise everywhere within the natural world. Observations and discussions can be made into things as fascinating as spider webs, leaf patterns, sunflowers and even coastlines. This makes math not only beautiful, but also inspiring and (dare we say) fun!

Pappas Method

For parents and teachers to assist their students in discovering the true wonders of mathematics, the techniques of Theoni Pappas can easily be applied, as per her popular and celebrated book "Fractals, Googols and Other Mathematical Tales." Pappas used to be a math phobia sufferer and created a fascinating step-by-step program for parents and teachers to use in order to teach students the joy of math.

Her simple, constructive step-by-step program goes as follows:

Don't let your fear of math come across to your kids - Parents must be careful not to perpetuate the mathematical myth - that math is only for specially talented "math types." Strive not to make comments like; "they don't like math" or "I have never been good at math." When children overhear comments like these from their primary role models they begin to dread math before even considering a chance of experiencing its wonders. It is important to encourage your children to read and explore the rich world of mathematics, and to practice mathematics without imparting negative biases.

Don't immediately associate math with computation (counting) - It is very important to realize that math is not just numbers and computations, but a realm of exciting ideas that touch every part of our lives -from making a telephone call to how the hair grows on someone's head. Take your children outside and point out real objects that display math concepts. For example, show them the symmetry of a leaf or angles on a building. Take a close look at the spirals in a spider web or intricate patterns of a snowflake.

Help your child understand why math is important - Math improves problem solving, increases competency and should be applied in different ways. It's the same as reading. You can learn the basics of reading without ever enjoying a novel. But, where's the excitement in that? With math, you could stop with the basics. But why when there is so much more to be gained by a fuller Understanding? Life is so much more enriching when we go beyond the basics. Stretch your children's minds to become involved in mathematics in ways that will not only be practical but also enhance their lives.

Make math as "hands on" as possible - Mathematicians participate in mathematics. To really experience math encourage your child to dig in and tackle problems in creative ways. Help them learn how to manipulate numbers using concrete references they understand as well as things they can see or touch. Look for patterns everywhere, explore shapes and symmetries. How many octagons do you see each day on the way to the grocery store? Play math puzzles and games and then encourage your child to try to invent their own. And, whenever possible, help your child realize a mathematical conclusion with real and tangible results. For example, measure out a full glass of juice with a measuring cup and then ask your child to drink half. Measure what is left. Does it measure half of a cup?

Read books that make math exciting:

Fractals, Googols and Other Mathematical Tales introduces an animated cat who explains fractals, tangrams and other mathematical concepts you've probably never heard of to children in terms they can understand. This book can double as a great text book by using one story per lesson.

A Wrinkle in Time is a well-loved classic, combining fantasy and science.

The Joy of Mathematics helps adults explore the beauty of mathematics that is all around.

The Math Curse is an amusing book for 4-8 year olds.

The Gnarly Gnews is a free, humorous bi-monthly newsletter on mathematics.

The Phantom Tollbooth is an Alice in Wonderland-style adventure into the worlds of words and numbers.

Use the internet to help your child explore the fascinating world of mathematics.

Web Math provides a powerful set of math-solvers that gives you instant answers to the stickiest problems.

Math League has challenging math materials and contests for fourth grade and above.

Silver Burdett Ginn Mathematics offers Internet-based math activities for grades K-6.

The Gallery of Interactive Geometry is full of fascinating, interactive geometry activities.

Math is very much like a language of its own. And like any second language, it will get rusty if it is not practiced enough. For that reason, students should always be looking into new ways to keep understanding and brushing up on their math skills, to be certain that foundations do not crumble, inhibiting the learning of new levels of math.

There are many different books, services and websites that have been developed to take the fear out of math, and to help even the most uncertain student develop self confidence in his or her math capabilities.

There is no reason for math or math classes to be a frightening experience, nor should it drive a student crazy, making them believe that they simply don't have the "math brain" that is needed to solve certain problems.

There are friendly ways to tackle such problems and it's all a matter of dispelling myths and creating a solid math foundation.

Concentrate on re-learning the basics and feeling better about yourself in math, and you'll find that the math brain you've always wanted, was there all along.

Special Report: Difficult Patients

Every nurse will eventually get a difficult patient on their list of responsibilities. These patients can be mentally, physically, and emotionally combative in many different environments. Consequently, care of these patients should be conducted in a manner for personal and self-protection of the nurse. Some of the key guidelines are as follows:

1. Never allow yourself to be cornered in a room with the patient positioned between you and the door.
2. Don't escalate the tension with verbal bantering. Basically, don't argue with the patient or resident.
3. Ask permission before performing any normal tasks in a patient's room whenever possible.
4. Discuss your concerns with other nursing staff. Consult the floor supervisor if necessary, especially when safety is an issue.
5. Get help from other support staff when offering care. Get a witness if you are anticipating abuse of any kind.
6. Remove yourself from the situation if you are concerned about your personal safety at all times.
7. If attacked, defend yourself with the force necessary for self-protection and attempt to separate from the patient.
8. Be aware of the patient's medical and mental history prior to entering the patient's room.
9. Don't put yourself in a position to be hurt.
10. Get the necessary help for all transfers, bathing and dressing activities from other staff members for difficult patients.
11. Respect the resident and patient's personal property.
12. Get assistance quickly, via the call bell or vocal projection, if a situation becomes violent or abuse.
13. Immediately seek medical treatment if injured.
14. Fill out an incident report for proper documentation of the occurrence.
15. Protect other patients from abusive behavior.

Special Report: Guidelines for Standard Precautions

Standard precautions are precautions taken to avoid contracting various diseases and preventing the spread of disease to those who have compromised immunity.

Some of these diseases include human immunodeficiency virus (HIV), acquired immunodeficiency syndrome (AIDS), and hepatitis B (HBV). Standard precautions are needed since many diseases do not display signs or symptoms in their early stages.

Standard precautions mean to treat all body fluids/ substances as if they were contaminated. These body fluids include but are not limited to the following blood, semen, vaginal secretions, breast milk, amniotic fluid, feces, urine, peritoneal fluid, synovial fluid, cerebrospinal fluid, secretions from the nasal and oral cavities, and lacrimal and sweat gland excretions.

This means that standard precautions should be used with all patients.

1. A shield for the eyes and face must be used if there is a possibility of splashes from blood and body fluids.
2. If possibility of blood or body fluids being splashed on clothing, you must wear a plastic apron.
3. Gloves must be worn if you could possibly come in contact with blood or body fluids. They are also needed if you are going to touch something that may have come in contact with blood or body fluids.
4. Hands must be washed even if you were wearing gloves. Hands must be washed and gloves must be changed between patients. Wash hands with at a dime size amount of soap and warm water for about 30 seconds. Singing "Mary had a little lamb" is approximately 30 seconds.
5. Blood and body fluid spills must be cleansed and disinfected using a solution of one part bleach to 10 parts water or your hospitals accepted method.
6. Used needles must be separated from clean needles. Throw both the needle and the syringe away in the sharps' container. The sharps' container is mad of puncture proof material.
7. Take extra care in performing high-risk activities that include puncturing the skin and cutting the skin.
8. CPR equipment to be used in a hospital must include resuscitation bags and mouthpieces.

Special precautions must be taken to dispose of biomedical waste. Biomedical waste includes but is not limited to the following laboratory waste, pathology waste, liquid waste from suction, all sharp object, bladder catheters, chest tubes, IV tubes, and drainage containers. Biomedical waste is removed from a facility by trained biomedical waste disposers.

The health care professional is legally and ethically responsible for adhering to standard precautions. They may prevent you from contracting a fatal disease or from a patient contracting a disease from you that could be deadly.

Special Report: Basic Review of Types of Fractures

A fracture is defined as a break in a bone that may sometimes involve cartilaginous structures. A fracture can be classified according to its cause or the type of break. The following definitions are used to describe breaks.

1. Traumatic fracture – break in a bone resulting from injury
2. Spontaneous fracture – break in a bone resulting from disease
3. Pathologic fracture – another name for a spontaneous fracture
4. Compound fracture – occurs when fracture bone is exposed to the outside by an opening in the skin
5. Simple fracture - occurs when a break is contained within the skin
6. Greenstick fracture - a traumatic break that is incomplete and occurs on the convex surface of the bend in the bone
7. Fissured fracture – a traumatic break that involves an incomplete longitudinal break
8. Comminuted fracture – a traumatic break that involves a complete fracture that results in several bony fragments
9. Transverse fracture – a traumatic break that is complete and occurs at a right angle to the axis of the bone
10. Oblique fracture- a traumatic break that occurs at an angle other than a right angel to the axis of the bone.
11. Spiral fracture – a traumatic break that occurs by twisting a bone with extreme force

A compound fracture is much more dangerous than a simple break. This is due to the break in skin that can allow microorganisms to infect the injured tissue. When a fracture occurs, blood vessels within the bone and its periosteum are disrupted. The periosteum, covering of fibrous connective tissue on the surface of the bone, may also be damaged or torn.

Special Report: Additional Bonus Material

Due to our efforts to try to keep this book to a manageable length, we've created a link that will give you access to all of your additional bonus material.

Please visit http://www.mometrix.com/bonus948/paxrn to access the information.